SCHERING

With compliments
Schering Diagnostics

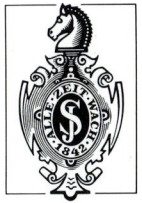

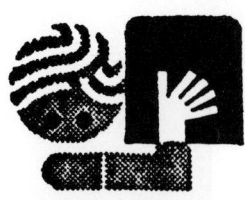 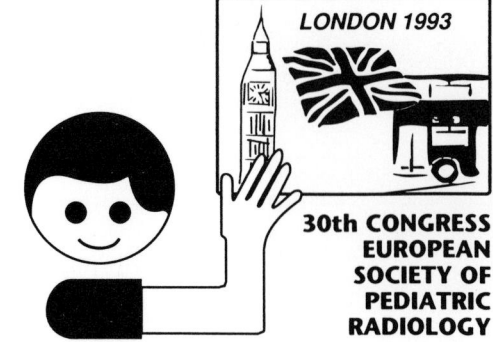

This emblem was first used by Dr. K. KNAPP at the Madrid meeting of the ESPR in 1975. It was subsequently adopted as the official logo of the society and a variation according to the location of the conference has been used since then.

Herbert J. Kaufmann
Hans Ringertz
Elisabeth Sweet
(Eds.)

The First 30 Years of the ESPR

The History of Pediatric Radiology in Europe

Springer-Verlag
Berlin Heidelberg New York
London Paris Tokyo
Hong Kong Barcelona
Budapest

Professor Dr. Herbert J. Kaufmann
Schwerinstr. 14
W-1000 Berlin 30, FRG

Professort Dr. Hans Ringertz
Karolinska Hospital, Department of Radiology
10401 Stockholm, Sweden

Elisabeth Sweet, M.D.
Royal Hospital for Sick Children, X-Ray Department
Glasgow G3 8SJ, United Kingdom

With 45 Figures and 2 Tables

ISBN 3-540-56541-8 Springer-Verlag Berlin Heidelberg New York
ISBN 0-387-56541-8 Springer-Verlag New York Berlin Heidelberg

This work is subject to copyright. All rights are reserved, whether the whole or part of the material is concerned, specifically the rights of translation, reprinting, reuse of illustrations, recitation, broadcasting, reproduction on microfilm or in other way, and storage in data banks. Duplication of this publication or parts thereof is permitted only under the provisions of the German Copyright Law of September 9, 1965, in its current version, and permission for use must always be obtained from Springer-Verlag. Violations are liable for prosecution under the German Copyright Law.

© Springer-Verlag Berlin Heidelberg 1993
Printed in Germany

The use of registered names, trademarks, etc. in this publication does not imply, even in the absence of a specific statement, that such names are exempt from the relevant protective laws and regulations and therefore free for general use.

Product liability: The publishers cannot guarantee the accuracy of any information about dosage and application contained in this book. In every individual case the user must check such information by consulting the relevant literature.

Typesetting, printing and bookbinding: Konrad Triltsch, Würzburg
21/3130-5 4 3 2 1 0 – Printed on acid-free paper

Preface

Our society is entering its fourth decade of existence, as of the 30th Annual Meeting in London, and we felt that this event merited reflection – a look back into the past – so as to better appreciate where we come from and where our subspeciality stands today, also in order to understand our colleagues from the different areas in Europe. It is our hope that paediatric radiology in Europe will thereby be strengthened now that old barriers have fallen.

At the second conjoint meeting of the ESPR and the SPR in Stockholm in 1991 a group of senior pediatric radiologists from all parts of Europe who felt that this occasion should be marked took the initiative to produce a book on the history of paediatric radiology focussing on the developments leading to the creation of the ESPR.

We thank all the colleagues who participated in the initial meeting to plan this book in Stockholm in 1991 and again at the Budapest Meeting in 1992 and who subsequently prepared contributions for it. These are the authors of the respective chapters and with them we hope that our readers will appreciate this effort. Unfortunately, we were not able to cover every European country, in spite of our attempt to do so.

Our sincere thanks go to Dr. Clauss and Dr. Renate Keysser-Götze of Schering, Berlin, who enthusiastically supported our plan to produce this book and also to Dr. Ute Heilmann of Springer-Verlag, Heidelberg. They were extremely supportive and generous so that this book can be presented to the participants of the London Meeting in 1993.

HERBERT J. KAUFMANN, HANS RINGERTZ and ELISABETH SWEET

Contents

General Introduction
H. J. KAUFMANN 1

Emergence of Pediatric Radiology in France
J. SAUVEGRAIN and C. FAURÉ 5

Development of Paediatric Radiology in Scandinavia and Finland
O. EKLÖF and U. RUDHE 17

Development of Pediatric Radiology in Austria
W. SWOBODA 27

The History of Pediatric Radiology in Czechoslovakia
S. TŮMA, E. KOLIHOVÁ and A. RUBÍN 29

The History of Paediatric Radiology in Germany
W. WILLICH and K.-D. EBEL 39

Paediatric Radiology in Great Britain and Ireland
E. SWEET 59

The History of Pediatric Radiology in Hungary
K. GEFFERTH, E. SCHLÄFFER and B. LOMBAY 69

Paediatric Radiology in Italy: Its Status Before and After
the Foundation of the European Society of Paediatric Radiology
G. BELUFFI 79

Paediatric Radiology in the Netherlands
P. P. G. KRAMER 93

Pediatric Radiology in Poland
A. Marciński 99

The History of Pediatric Radiology in Romania
M. Radulescu 109

Pediatric Radiology in Spain
V. Pérez-Candela and J. Lucaya 111

The History of Pediatric Radiology in Switzerland
A. Giedion 113

List of Contributors

BELUFFI, G., M.D., Policlinico San Matteo, Servizio di Radiodiagnostica, Piazzale Golgi, I-27100 Pavia

EBEL, K.-D., Prof. Dr., Birkenweg 3, W-5000 Köln 40, FRG

EKLÖF, O., M.D., Karolinska Hospital, Department of Radiology, P.O. Box 65000, S-10401 Stockholm

FAURÉ, C., Prof., Hôpital Trousseau, 8-28 Avenue du Dr. Arnold Netter, F-75571 Paris

GEFFERTH, K., Doz. † (died 1992)

GIEDION, A., Prof. Dr., Doldertal 7, CH-8032 Zürich

KAUFMANN, H.J., Prof. Dr., Schwerinstr. 14, W-1000 Berlin 30, FRG

KOLIHOVÁ, E., Dr., Faculty Hospital Motol, V. Uvalu 84, 15018 Praha 5, Czech Republic

KRAMER, P.P.G., M.D., University Hospital for Children and Youth, Het Wilhelmina Kinderziekenhuis, P.O. Box 18009, NL-3501 CA Utrecht

LOMBAY, B., M.D., Child Health Center, Department of Radiology, H-3501 Miskolc Szentpeteri Kapu 76

LUCAYA, J., M.D., Hospital Infantil, Department of Radiology, Valle Hebron, E-08035 Barcelona

MARCIŃSKI, A., M.D., Department of Pediatric Radiology, Children's Hospital of the Medical Academy, Marshallkowska, P-04-736 Warszawa

PÉREZ-CANDELA, V., Dr., Centro Medico de Radiodiagnostico, Garcia Tello 7, E-35016 Las Palmas de Gran Canaria

RADULESCU, M., Dr., Spitalul Clinic de Copii "Maria Sklodowska Curie", B-dul C. Brincoveanu Nr. 20, Sector 4, cod. 755544, Bucharest, Romania

List of Contributors

RUBÍN, A., Prof., Detska A Dorostova, Klinika FVL UK, Ke Karlovu, 12109 Praha 2, Czech Republic

RUDHE, U., M.D., Huddinge Sjukhus, Department of Radiology, S-14186 Huddinge

SAUVEGRAIN, J., Prof., 202 Avenue du Maine, F-75014 Paris

SCHLÄFFER, E., Dr., Julia U. 2cI5, H-1015 Budapest

SWEET, E., M.D., Royal Hospital for Sick Children, X-Ray Department, UK-G3 8SJ Glasgow

SWOBODA, W., Prof. Dr., Schwarzspanierstr. 11, A-1090 Vienna

TŮMA, S., Dr., Paediatric Cardio Center, University Hospital Motol, 15018 Praha 5, Czech Republic

WILLICH, E., Prof. Dr., Sitzbuchweg 20, W-6900 Heidelberg, FRG

General Introduction

H. J. Kaufmann

When the Society for Pediatric Radiology (SPR) celebrated its 25th anniversary, the occasion was marked by a booklet commemorating the origins and its founders and included personal recollections of the circumstances of its coming into existence in 1958. When our society reached its 25th year during the eminently successful Montreux meeting splendidly organized by Daniel Nusslé, this date unfortunately went unmarked. Therefore it is high time to record some historical facts and events that led to the foundation of the European Society of Paediatric Radiology (ESPR) and to focus on the origins of paediatric radiology in the different European countries. The London meeting in 1993, the 30th anniversary of the ESPR, appears to be the logical moment to put together such a book of historical sketches. At the international congress of paediatric radiology in Stockholm, the Co-President Hans Ringertz and the Secretary General Gabriel Kalifa immediately supported this idea and a meeting was organized bringing together the prospective authors. At that time we discussed the matter and it was felt that the focus should be on the early developments of paediatric radiology in the different countries with reference to the period prior to and at the time of foundation of the ESPR. When the group met again in Budapest in 1992, the manuscript on Scandinavia by O. Eklöf and U. Rudhe was distributed as an outline.

When in 1963 the international meeting of paediatric radiology took place in Paris, the foundation was laid for creating the ESPR with individual membership from all countries throughout Europe. At that time, there were no national organizations of paediatric radiologists and the links between individuals actively engaged in paediatric radiology had to be established by personal initiative, direct contacts at radiological and paediatric meetings and by simply "reaching out" to stimulate potentially interested colleagues to participate. The initial spark came unquestionably from Paris. The problem at that time simply was to determine who was to be approached and how to get the right people together.

In the fall of 1960, when I had just started my fellowship at his department in Boston, E. B. D. Neuhauser asked me one morning, "Herb, do you know French?" When I promptly answered, "yes", he was visibly relieved, telling me we were expecting a prominent visitor the following week who hardly spoke English. He was referring to J. Lefèbvre, whom I had the pleasure of getting to know through daily contact for 2 weeks, first in Boston and subsequently in Atlantic City at the annual meeting of the combined American Roentgen-ray Society and SPR meeting. After my return to Basel in 1961, an invitation arrived from Paris to participate in a meeting on skeletal dysplasias with the main speakers P. Rubin and P. Maroteaux. At the international paediatric meeting in Lisbon in 1962, J. Lefèbvre initiated a dinner meeting at a restaurant "Cavallo Branco" attended amongst others by F. N. Silverman, Cl. Fauré, A. Lassrich and myself. There he proposed the idea of an international meeting just for paediatric radiologists in Paris the following year. All those present gave enthusiastic support and did their best to activate colleagues in their regions interested in our field. This solid groundwork by the Paris group – J. Lefèbvre, J. Sauvegrain and Cl. Fauré – was eminently successful as can be seen in the following articles.

A special aspect of our society has to do with the "use of languages". Both at the initial Paris meeting and at the London meeting French and English were accepted as official congress languages. At the second meeting in Stockholm German was also accepted. At the Basel meeting in 1967, since German was the local language, simultaneous translation was provided not only for two but for three languages. The cost for this simply got out of hand and, furthermore, the quality was not particularly good. Since in our society a number of people are multilingual, I argued at the meeting of the officers of the ESPR in the fall of 1966 that we should limit our meetings to one language, English. This was a very difficult step for our French friends to take. However, for the sake of a healthy development of the society and to contain the costs of the meetings, this was not only accepted but J. Lefèbvre put great effort into learning English properly, setting an example which was followed by our French colleagues and others who then were not yet in full command of that language. Therefore, beginning with the Hamburg meeting in 1968, this was no longer a "problem". It should, however, be added that on the evening of the mentioned officers' meeting in Paris, J. Lefèbvre told my wife "Anita, *votre mari est méchant*" (Anita, your husband is wicked), but this in no way affected our friendship! In those early years of our society, many bonds were established across national borders and language barriers and those fortunate to have been part of the initial phase of our society's creation considered each other simply as part of "the family".

Under the guidance of J. Lefèbvre and E. B. D. Neuhauser the groundwork was laid for the publication of a book series "Progress in Paediatric Radiology" and an editorial committee formed. With the help of R. Astley, G. Currarino, S. Dunbar, C. Fauré, U. Rudhe and F. N. Silverman, seven volumes were produced from 1967 to 1980. At the time these served well and many of the articles from all over the world have become landmarks. Due to the advent of our speciality journal *Paediatric Radiology* the series was discontinued. The first three volumes were translated into Spanish by K. Knapp.

During my training period at the Boston City Hospital in the late 1950s, I had a chance meeting on the way to one of the famous CPC's organized by Castleman at the Massachusetts General Hospital. The speaker was Prof. Ühlinger, the well-known bone pathologist from Zurich. On the narrow winding stairway to the auditorium it became obvious to me that the tall slender person walking next to me was also a young physician from Switzerland. As it turned out, this was Andres Giedion, whom I subsequently visited at the Boston Children's Hospital. In those days Boston was the "Mecca of medicine" but particularly the department of E. B. D. Neuhauser, the "leading light of paediatric radiology".

The impact of this institution and of the then budding SPR can clearly be recognized in this book. The initial articles are those from France and Scandinavia. The first one, written by J. Sauvegrain and C. Fauré, relates how the ESPR came into existence. The following contribution by O. Eklöf and U. Rudhe documents clearly why and how in Sweden and subsequently emanating from there radiology as a diagnostic speciality and consequently also paediatric radiology had taken an uncontestable place. That paediatric radiology has still not received academic recognition, however, is, to say the least, "unfortunate". The rest of the contributions are presented in alphabetical order. All authors were aware of the content of the article on Scandinavia as a suggested format. Each article is the expression of local, national, linguistic and particularly personal characteristics of the individual author(s). Some presentations are short, sketchy and tensely written, some more extensive, occasionally containing anecdotes. The contribution from Germany relates the developments in the light of the separation of the country, where from 1949 as the consequence of the post-war situation two countries existed for 40 years. This brings us to the dramatic political changes which have occurred in Europe since 1989. During the days of the "iron curtain" one special purpose of our society was clear – to bring together paediatric radiologists from all European countries. This was already possible at the initial meeting in Paris in 1963 and in 1964 and particularly when the meeting was held in a non-NATO country such as Sweden or Switzerland. At the Basel meeting in 1967 a delegation of eight Russian paediatric radiologists attended. In those days organizing the ESPR meeting was a very personal task and to invite participants from the former socialist countries meant going through a lot of red tape and finding the needed funding. Looking back, it is gratifying to see that in spite of the existing obstacles contacts could be established and maintained with paediatric radiologists from Eastern Europe. Regrettably in this book no contribution could be obtained from Russia, Bulgaria or, understandably, the former Yugoslavia. On the other hand, Poland, the Czech Republic, Slovakia and Rumania as well as Hungary and the former German Democratic Republic are well covered.

The manuscript from Hungary – where we had such a wonderful congress in Budapest in 1992 – will stand out. The first part on the historical aspects was written by Károly Gefferth. For all the participants at the Budapest meeting it was simply astonishing to see and hear this elder statesman of paediatric radiology and observe his perfect gentlemanly manners – a last glimpse at the style and culture of the former Austro-Hungarian Empire. He wrote his contribution in 1991. Six months after the Budapest meeting he passed away. He actually prepared two manuscripts, a short version which is included here and a longer one which will be published by Dr. Lombay in the "Yearbook of Paediatric Radiology". In Budapest he showed me his sketchbook containing two faithful drawings he made of his "X-ray laboratory" in 1954 (p. 71). Other sketches depicted his vineyard in the countryside near Budapest where he tended his wines up to his last year of life. At a visit to his home years ago, he proudly got a wonderfully aged bottle of his own wine out of his cellar.

We can only hope and wish that paediatric radiology in Europe will have a similarly long and rewarding career as our honorary member Károly Gefferth, a man who will not be forgotten by any of us. With the kind permission of Prof. H.-R. Wiedemann, Kiel, a reprint from the *European Journal of Paediatrics* devoted to Károly Gefferth in the series "The pioneers of paediatric medicine" follows the Hungarian contribution.

Emergence of Pediatric Radiology in France

J. SAUVEGRAIN and C. FAURÉ

In France some departments of pediatrics are housed in a general hospital. However, in many cities some hospitals are entirely devoted to children; in Paris there are five: Saint-Vincent de Paul, Trousseau, les Enfants-Malades, Robert Debré, and Bicêtre. This is also true in other cities: e.g., "hopital des Enfants" in Bordeaux, Saint-Charles in Montpellier, Debrousse in Lyon, Bretonneau in Tours, Charles Nicolle in Rouen, and Jeanne d'Arc in Vandoeuvre les Nancy.

In the early 1940s, all of these pediatric hospitals had a department of electroradiology. Electrotherapy was the main activity of these departments. Fluoroscopic examinations of the thorax, heart, mediastinum, and upper GI tract were done by pediatricians, surgeons, and/or radiologists. Babies were introduced into a bag hung behind the vertical fluoroscopic screen. Radiographs made by technicians were of poor quality, due to poor equipment and lack of appropriate devices to immobilize patients. The films were interpreted by pediatricians.

However, some basic elements of a pediatric X-ray department were already present. Radiologists were reponsible for the X-ray machines and for protecting the patients against radiation hazards. They had the opportunity to become pediatric radiologists, but most of them spent only a few months, at most 1 or 2 years, in a children's hospital; they did not become involved in pediatric radiodiagnosis but waited for a position as radiologist in a hospital for adults where they expected to find more cooperative patients and diseases they were familiar with.

Some changes occurred in 1942–1943: at the Enfants-Malades, fluoroscopy of the chest and upper GI tract was performed in the Pediatric Department only by a radiologist, E. Mignon, who had experience in pediatrics. At Saint-Vincent de Paul Hospital there was a pediatrician, M. Lelong, whose department handled a large number of premature births and neonates; an outstanding surgeon, P. Petit; and an inventive radiologist, M. Aymé. To examine newborns and infants, Aymé designed a device which immobilized these patients efficiently and comfortably. The device was easily fixed on any existing vertical or horizontal tilting radiology table. Rarely has such a simple and cheap device been as useful as "la Roue d'Aymé".

Just after World War II, J. Barnard and R. Lebouchard turned their attention to the technical aspects of radiography of infants and children; H. Fischgold and C. Juster made an interesting anatomoradiological correlation of bone growth. But Jacques Lefèbvre, was the first to make pediatric radiology his main, lifelong interest. He started his residency in 1934, working with leading people of that time in radiology: L. Delherm, L. Gally, P. Porcher, and L. Mallet. He was elected to the "Bureau Central" in 1947 and became chief Radiologist of the Department of Radiology of "Les Enfants-Malades" in 1948. He remained there until his death in 1974.

When Lefèbvre arrived in 1948, 70 beds in the hospital were devoted to diagnosis and treatment of patients with poliomyelitis; this was the era prior to the availability of vaccination. The department of Electroradiology was in charge of electrodiagnosis and electrotherapy of these patients. J. Lefèbvre had his consulting room in an old but large building. In contrast, the area devoted to radiodiagnosis did not exceed 100 m^2 and was located in the basement of the far-removed pediatric surgery building.

The leaders of the hospital were very well known pediatricians: Robert Debré, Maurice Lamy, Jean Bernard and their associates, P. Royer, P. Mozziconacci, J. Gerbeaux, S. Thieffry, and Julien Marie, whose notoriety ensured an outstanding number of admissions to the hospital. In surgery, H. Leveuf initiated the separation of visceral surgery from orthopedics; this development was completed by M. Fèvre, J. Judet, B. Duhamel, and D. Pellerin. The achievements in pediatric surgery were superb. For radiology this environment was stimulating and challenging!

Until 1939, French was an accepted language in medicine, as were German and English. After a 6-year hiatus, penicillin became available from the United Kingdom; radiology (and medicine in general) now expressed itself in English. Truth came from Sweden through the *Acta Radiologica Scandinavica*. Radiodiagnosis was separating from radiotherapy. Cerebral angiography and angiocardiography had been developed. The second Symposium Neuroradiologicum was held in Rotterdam in 1949, the third one in Stockholm in 1952. In the same year, Clément Fauré spent 4 months at the Karolinska Institute; he was succeeded the following year by Jean Bennet. The International Congress took place in Copenhagen in 1953. Everybody was impressed by Scandinavian achievements in radiology. F. J. Hodges, an American radiologist and one of the Year Book reviewers, wrote a special article about this phenomenon (*One American's View of Scandinavian Radiology*, Year Book of Radiology, Chicago 1954–1955 series, pp 7–11).

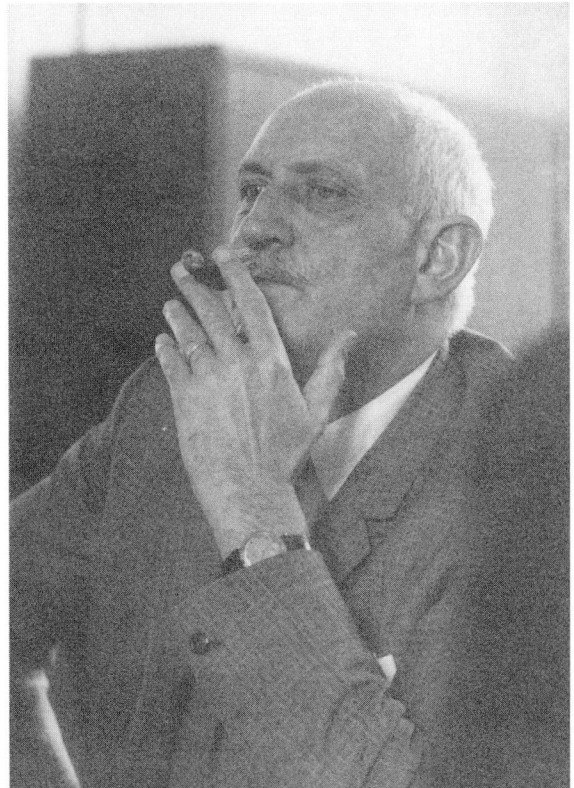

Figure 1
Prof. J. Lefèbvre, the father of the ESPR

At that time, Jacques Lefèbvre had only a few people working with him: Jean Lerique in Electrology, Antoinette Lerique for EEG. For Radiodiagnosis, he had E. Guy, R. Leisner, and J. Sauvegrain, soon to be joined by Clément Fauré. Later on, "younger people" were enrolled: J. Bennet, P. Chaumont, M. Fortier-Beaulieu, J. Le Gall, and G. Di Chiro, among others. Very quickly we were involved in all medical and surgical staff meetings at the hospital: we assumed responsibility for the wards, the emergency services, and for mutual teaching. The atmosphere of the department was busy, studious, and cheerful. Contact was established with radiologists of other pediatric hospitals: C. Béraud and P. Deffrenne, Lyon; P. Jouve, Marseille; P. Guichard, Bordeaux; M. Bretagne, Nancy; A. Wackenheim, Strassbourg. The department trained radiologists who would be in charge at pediatric hospitals in the 1960s, general radiologists

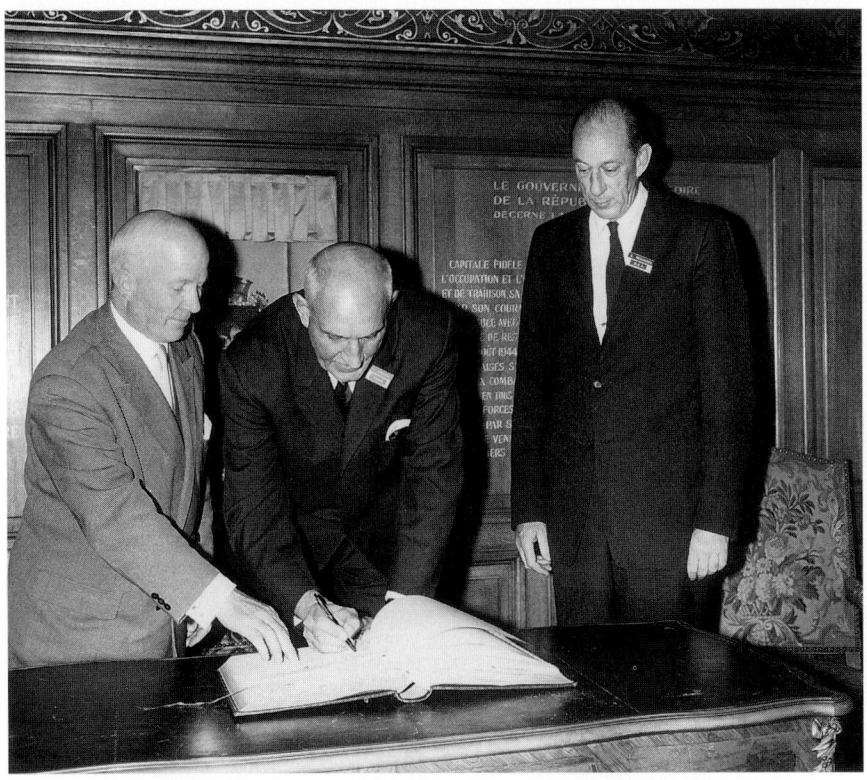

Figure 2
J. Lefèbvre signing the Golden Book of the City of Paris and E. B. D. Neuhauser waiting his turn. Reception in the City Hall at the International Meeting in Paris 1963

who worked part time in pediatric radiology, or general radiologists interested in "clinical" and not only "technical radiology".

At the same time, the wind was also blowing from the West: the first edition of John Caffey's book (Year Book Publishers, Chicago) appeared in 1945, the second in 1950. "The Book", as we called it in the department, was our first reference work (and has remained so). We surveyed articles published in pediatric, surgical, or radiological journals. Progress in radiology resulted from progress in medical knowledge or in imaging technology; these advances took place on both sides of the Atlantic.

In 1957, J. Lefèbvre visited Ed Neuhauser at the Children's Hospital in Boston, J. Caffey at Babies' Hospital in New York, and Scott Dunbar at Montreal Children's Hospital. He was impressed by the establishment of radiology in USA, similar (but less contracted) to the situation in Sweden.

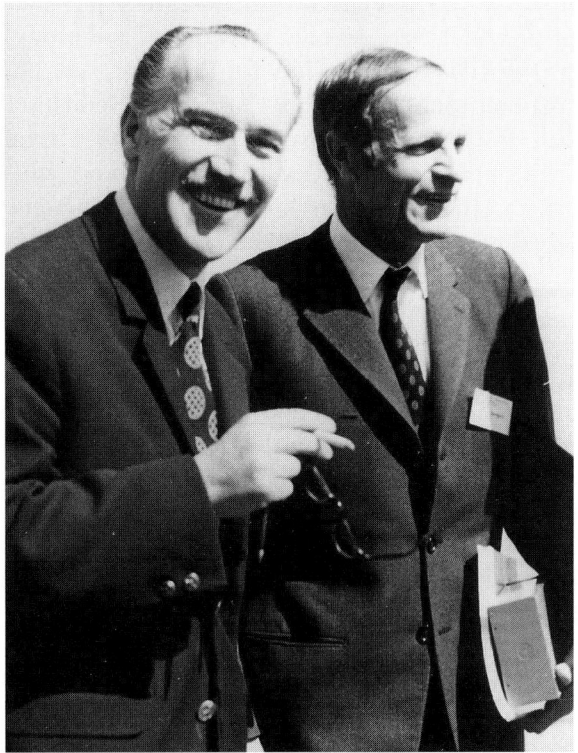

Figure 3
C. Fauré and J. Sauvegrain, past presidents and secretaries of the ESPR (1972 J. S., 1983 C. F.) relaxing during the Hamburg meeting in 1968

He was fascinated by the number, the seriousness, and the quality of American pediatric radiologists, and by the broad acceptance that pediatric radiology enjoyed.

In 1958, Lefèbvre published, in a new journal, *Annales de Radiologie*, an editorial dedicated to pediatric radiology.

Pediatric radiology concerns the entirety of radiodiagnosis (we should say now "imaging") in normal as well as in sick children. Pediatric radiology is a subspeciality of radiology justified by diseases or peculiar presentation of diseases in patients of pediatric age. . . . Pediatric radiology is not characterized by size or non-participation of the patients but by peculiarities of diseases affecting a differentiating or growing organism. . . . The pediatric radiologist must always keep in mind that the dynamic organism of the child is more sensible than any other to the aggressiveness of X-rays. . . . In pediatrics, to lose time entails the risk of losing a life, or permanent disability for an entire life. . . . Radiologists who perform children's examinations must be well-informed and competent.

This editorial was an Introduction to the *Journées Nationales de Radiologie* 1958, one day of which was devoted to pediatric radiology.

In the same year, 1958, the Society for Pediatric Radiology (SPR) was founded in Washington D. C. John Caffey, E. Neuhauser, A. Tucker, F. N. Silverman, B. Girdany, S. Ross, J. Gwinn and G. Currarino were not myths, but living persons, intellectually curious about what you do and how you do it, and they were ready to share their experience. Here, as in France, it seemed necessary to strengthen pediatric radiology with regard to adult radiology, hospital management, and university authorities. The SPR as a scientific society established pediatric radiology as a subspecialty of radiology.

Each year, one or several French radiologists participated in the annual meeting of the SPR. We had the opportunity to meet there E. Singleton, J. Kirkpatrick, G. Harris, W. Berdon, J. Baker, J. Hope, and R. Lester. We were not the only Europeans to attend the SPR meetings, we met or we heard of many distinguished European colleagues: R. Astley, J. Sutcliffe, S. R. Kjellberg, U. Rudhe, P. Franklin, A. Giedion, H. J. Kaufmann, G. Iannaccone, D. Nusslé, L. G. Blair, W. Holthusen, H. Fendel, A. Lassrich, K. Rowinski, and many others.

The idea of a sister society in Europe was in the air. The team from Paris proposed and organized an informal preliminary meeting in Paris in 1963, with the help of the SPR, to explore the feasibility. The meeting was successful. The European Society for Pediatric Radiology (ESPR) held its first meeting in 1964 in Paris, with J. Lefèbvre as its first president, again with a massive attendance by members of the SPR.

The statutes of the new society were resolutely European and were well accepted and applied. Thereafter the development of pediatric radiology in each European country was more or less interconnected with that of the ESPR. The adoption of English as the official language (Basel, 1967) facilitated the "growing together" of this European community. Later on, French- and German-speaking groups of pediatric radiologists were founded, affiliated with their respective national radiological societies. These groups work efficiently with, not against, the ESPR to spread knowledge about pediatric radiology throughout the respective linguistic communities.

Editorial

(International Reunion of Pediatric Radiologists, May 1963)
Soon after Roentgen's discovery, paediatric radiology took a brilliant start with the publication in 1898 of Escherich's article on the value of radiography for diagnosis in children (La

valeur diagnostique de la radiographie chez l'enfant). However, for over 30 years, its development lagged behind that of both general radiology and paediatrics.

The reason for it was one of equipment. Now that this has been solved, the very precise techniques used previously for adults only can be applied to children as well, and since 1930, a remarkable series of prominent works has been published, bearing names such as those of Caffey, Neuhauser in the U.S.A., Blair in England, Schall in Germany, Kjellberg in Sweden.

Radiopediatrics as a new branch of medicine was applied at times by paediatricians, at other times by radiologists. It gradually became autonomous, as shown by the setting up in the U.S.A. of the American Society for Paediatric Radiology in 1958. During the last 5 years, the increasing importance of this society's annual meetings and the value of the works described on such occasions have more than justified its existence.

Our present meeting is held under the aegis of both the International Children's Center (Centre International de l'Enfance) and the European Association of Radiology. Such a twofold sponsorship is a clear indication of now essential it is for paediatrics as well as radiology to be closely combined in the training of radiopaediatricians. It is our hope that the meeting will respond to the wishes expressed by radiopaediatricians at previous international gatherings on radiology and paediatrics, and in particular that it will provide the necessary basis for the setting up of a European Society for Paediatric Radiology.

Many radiologists have come over from America to join us. We thank them for their active cooperation. Their experience will be most helpful in constituting our own group. Their presence is a proof of the friendly links which will unite our societies on both sides of the ocean.

We would like to express our gratitude to the members of the Executive Board of the International Children's Center, in particular to its Chairman, Professor Robert Debré, who have kindly put at our disposal the premises and facilities of the Center in this beautiful castle of Longchamp. We also thank Doctor Berthet, Director General or the I.C.C. who has done his utmost to help us, Doctor Sauvegrain and Doctor Fauré, whose devoted work has made it possible to hold this meeting, and finally to Mlle Fachard, the key organizer of our Secretariat.

J. Lefèbvre

Editorial

(First Session of the ESPR, May 1964)
The European Society of Pediatric Radiologists was founded at the time of the International Reunion held in 1963 at the Château de Longchamp with the warm collaboration of the American Society for Pediatric Radiology. You will find further on the text of the statutes which have been drawn up by the committee named for this purpose.

In the text a distinction is made between the active members and associate members. This distinction merites an explanation. It appeared to us preferable that the Pediatric Radiologist be at the same time exclusively radiologist and pediatrician, in our society the title of active member is reserved for those who practice pediatric radiology exclusively.

This exists on a large scale in the U.S.A., Great Britain and Poland. This is beginning to develop in France (at Paris and Lyon), in Switzerland (at Basel and Lausanne), in Germany (at Hamburg) and in Sweden (at Stockholm). But in many European cities it is still the general radiologist who examines the hospitalized children, devoting only a part of his time to our discipline. The general radiologist who devotes part of his time to Pediatric Radiology will be eligible for an associate membership the same as the pediatric surgeons or pediatricians who are interested in radiology.

It is one of the essential goals of our association to demonstrate the necessity for the individualization of the discipline of Pediatric Radiology and to see that individualization obtained throughout Europe. Wherever there are Pediatricians or Pediatric surgeons, there ought to be a Pediatric radiologist.

The first meeting of the European Society opens on a happy note with the presence of five of our American colleagues who have again honored us with their presence. The European participants are more numerous than last year; the number of presentations and their interest have again this year obliged us to extend the duration of the meeting to two and a half days.

The communications cover most of the actual fields of interest of Pediatric Radiology. Nearly one day will be devoted to the important problem of the acute abdomen of the infant. Subjects included in these sessions under the direction of Pr. Lassrich are: neonatal obstruction, volvulus, perforation, Hirschprung disease, and Henoch-Schoenlein purpura.

We would like to thank at this time the Centre International de l'Enfance for the welcome offered us here at the Château de Longchamp with its intimate atmosphere so suitable for this type of meeting.

Aided by our experience with the meeting of 1963 we have avoided certain errors but we hope that those technical imperfections which will no doubt arise this time will pass unnoticed among the general feeling of good will and enthousiasm of each of you.

Our secretaires Dr. Sauvegrain and Fauré have not been sparing of their time or patience. Miss Fachard, Mrs Delong and Miss Sartori are at the disposition of each of you to help resolve any menu problems which may occur during the course of your stay in a foreign city; that is the most agreeable part of their job.

This reunion confirms the autonomy of our discipline within the framework of Pediatrics and Radiology. My thanks to all of you who are participating here.

Dr. J. Lefèbvre

Statutes of the European Society of Pediatric Radiology

The purposes of the European Society of Pediatric Radiology are:
  1. To organize and bring together pediatric radiologists
  2. To contribute to the progress of Pediatric Radiology in the European countries in conjunction with the other sectors of Radiology and Pediatrics, as much in the clinical and scientific domains as in that which concerns education and teaching

In order to realize these goals, the Society can:
  1. Organize European congresses, sessions and conferences;
  2. Cooperate with the Society for Pediatric Radiology and the European Association of Radiology as well as with other scientific organizations

The Society is nonprofit, nonsecular, and nonpolitical.

The Members

The Society consists of active members, associate members, honorary members, and corresponding members.

The Active Members of the European Society of Pediatric Radiology are limited to those persons possessing the Diploma of Doctor of Medicine, authorized to practice medicine, and whose principal activity is Pediatric Radiology.

The active members are chosen by co-optation; their number shall not exceed 100.

The Associate Members can be chosen from among pediatricians or pediatric surgeons who are interested in certain areas of pediatric radiology and general radiologists who devote part of their activity to pediatric radiology. Their nomination will be confirmed by a simple majority of the active members meeting in a General Assembly.

The *Corresponding Members* are chosen by the General Assembly from pediatric radiologists working or residing outside of Europe.

The title of *Honory Member* is awarded by a General Assembly of active members in recognition of and as a singular distinction to those persons who have contributed significantly to progress in and the knowledge of pediatric radiology.

Governing Procedures

Officers

The officers include a President, two Vice Presidents, a Corresponding Secretary, a Secretary-Treasurer: these officers are elected by the General Assembly for three years; each year, the first Vice President succeeds to the presidency at the beginning of the annual reunion; at the same time the second Vice President succeeds to the office of first Vice President. Thus, each year a second Vice President is elected.

The officers are the administrators of the Society.

Committees

A certain number of committees are to be created within the Society, in particular a Committee of Candidature which will include as nearly as possible a member from each European country, and a Committee of Accounts to review the books and reports of the Secretary-Treasurer.

Meetings

An annual meeting of the Society will be held in Europe, the place and the date to be announced at least three months before the reunion.

The Reunion will consist of a General Assembly, which will make all decisions concerning the function of the Society. The decisions will be reached by a simple majority of the active members with a quorum of one third.

Revenues

The revenues of the Society will consist of contributions, gifts, legacies, subsidies, dues of the active members and associate members, and all other resources authorized by law.

The annual dues will be fixed by the General Assembly. The dues are payable on January 1 of each year.

Duration and Dissolution

The Society is constituted for an unlimited duration. Its dissolution can be pronounced only by the General Assembly by a vote of two thirds of the active members present.

J. Sauvegrain and C. Fauré

Honorary Members of the Society

John Caffey (USA)	1964
Lutz Schall (Germany)	1964
Sven Roland Kjellberg (Sweden)	1965
Edward B. D. Neuhauser (USA)	1965
Jacques Lefèbvre (France)	1966
Karoly M. Gefferth (Hungary)	1973
Ksawery Rowinski (Poland)	1973
Frederic N. Silverman (USA)	1974
Ulf Rudhe (Sweden)	1975
John A. Kirkpatrick, Jr (USA)	1979
Arnold Lassrich (Germany)	1979
Jacques Sauvegrain (France)	1979
Clément Fauré (France)	1982
Andres Giedion (Switzerland)	1982
Eberhard Willich (Germany)	1983
Roy Astley (United Kingdom)	1984
Jean Bennet (France)	1987
Ole Eklöf (Sweden)	1987
Charles A. Gooding (USA)	1987
Derek Harwood-Nash (Canada)	1987
John Holt (USA)	1987
Andrew K. Poznanski (USA)	1987
Hooshang Taybi (USA)	1987
Herbert J. Kaufmann (Germany)	1988
Bryan Cremin (South Africa)	1989
Klaus-Dietrich Ebel (Germany)	1989
Helmut Fendel (Germany)	1989
Elisabeth M. Sweet (United Kingdom)	1989
Beverly Wood (USA)	1990
Edmund A. Franken (USA)	1990
Daniel Nusslé (Switzerland)	1990
Alan Crispin (United Kingdom)	1990
Walter Berdon (USA)	1992

Past Presidents and Meeting Sites of the ESPR

1964	Jacques Lefèbvre	Paris, France
1965	Ulf Rudhe	Stockholm, Sweden
1966	John Sutcliffe	London, United Kingdom
1967	Herbert J. Kaufmann	Basel, Switzerland
1968	Arnold Lassrich	Hamburg, Germany
1969	Ksawery Rowinski	Warsaw, Poland
1970	Guido Iannaccone	Rome, Italy
1971	Gregers Thomsen	Copenhagen, Denmark
1972	Jacques Sauvegrain	Paris, France
1973	Roy Astley	Birmingham, United Kingdom
1974	Per-Erik Heikel	Helsinki, Finland
1975	Klaus Knapp	Madrid, Spain
1976	Ole Eklöf	Stockholm, Sweden
1977	Andres Giedion	Luzern, Switzerland
1978	Noemi Perlmutter-Cremer	Brussels, Belgium
1979	Klaus-Dietrich Ebel	Cologne, Germany
1980	The Dutch Group of Pediatric Radiologists	The Hague, The Netherlands
1981	Gunnar Stake	Oslo, Norway
1982	Antonin Rubin	Prague, Czechoslovakia
1983	Clément C. Fauré	Paris, France
1984	Gian Franco Vichi	Florence, Italy
1985	Elizabeth Sweet	Glasgow, Scottland
1986	Javier Lucaya	Barcelona, Spain
1987	Denis Lallemand (ESPR) IPR Derek Harwood-Nash (SRP)	Toronto, Canada
1988	Daniel Nusslé	Montreux, Switzerland
1989	Noel Blake	Dublin, Ireland
1990	Helmut Fendel	Munich, Germany
1991	Hans Ringertz (ESPR) IPR Donald R. Kirks (SPR)	Stockholm, Sweden
1992	Bela Lombay	Budapest, Hungary
1993	Donald Shaw	London, United Kingdom

Development of Paediatric Radiology in Scandinavia and Finland

O. Eklöf and U. Rudhe

Denmark

Denmark belongs to the few countries in Europe without full-time positions for paediatric radiologists. The examinations are still performed by general radiologists, many of them, however, with special interest in paediatric radiology. This particularly applies to the University Hospitals of Copenhagen (KAS Gentofte, KAS Glostrup, Hvidovre Hospital, and Rikshospitalet), Odense, Aalborg and Aarhus and, to a lesser extent to four Central (County) Hospitals. Paediatrics, but in particular paediatric surgery, mainly is centralized in the University Hospitals.

In spite of this organization, Danish radiologists early contributed significantly to the science. Thus, J. M. Nordentoft had a special interest in hydrostatic reduction of bowel intussusception as early as in 1939. This was followed by several reports on large series of cases [14].

G. Thomsen, professor of diagnostic radiology at Rigshospitalet and president of the ESPR Meeting in Helsingör, 1971, was actively involved in paediatric research work. Among his contributions to science, an investigation on hiatus hernia in children deserves special attention [18]. Thomsen also was instrumental in stimulating colleagues to devote themselves to paediatric radiology. Among those who became interested in our profession in the early years, T. Rosendahl, M. Egeblad, M. Eiken, F. Galatius-Jensen, E. Rostgaard-Christensen, and J. Jensen may be mentioned. During the late 1950s and early 1960s, S. Brünner, elected professor of diagnostic radiology in Copenhagen in 1971, devoted himself to paediatric radiology. He and associated authors published about 20 papers on different topics [3, 4].

Founding Members of the ESPR were S. Brünner, A. R. Christensen, E. R. Christensen, M. Eiken, B. Petersen, and T. Rosendahl. The Danish Society of Paediatric Radiology was established in 1991 under the chairmanship of M. Egeblad.

O. Eklöf and U. Rudhe

Finland

Up to 1946, when a new Children's Hospital was inaugurated in Helsinki, paediatricians or general radiologists performed and interpreted necessary radiological examinations. P.-E. Heikel (Fig. 1), a founding Member of ESPR and President at the ESPR Meeting in Helsingfors/Helsinki in 1974,

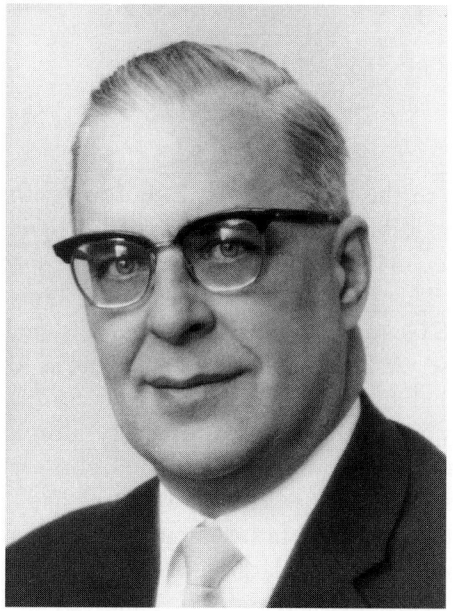

Figure 1
P.-E. Heikel, Finland

served for 5 years voluntarily as unpaid director of the radiology department in this hospital. During his early years as a paediatric radiologist he had widened his experience by visiting the radiological departments at the Samaritan Children's Hospital (acting radiologist: S. R. Kjellberg) and the Crown Princess Louise Children's Hospital (Head: F. Ulfsparre) in Stockholm. As a consequence of the latter visit he was able to introduce angiocardiography in his department. For more than two decades Heikel was sole chief radiologist in the subspeciality in Finland, bearing the brunt of the burden of training paediatric radiologists in the country. He also was scientifically active. He published some 15 papers on various topics [9].

During the 1970s and later on, positions as heads of newly created sections for paediatric radiology were established at all Finnish University Hospitals. First among this second generation of paediatric radiologists were E. Mäkinen of Turku and P. Lanning of Oulu, who both received part of their training at Karolinska Sjukhuset. It may also be mentioned that R. Stenström, director of the general radiology department of Aurora Hospital in Helsinki, practised paediatric radiology as well [17].

Paediatric Radiology in Finland has been an approved subspeciality since 1969. The Finnish Society of Paediatric Radiology, founded in the early 1980s, is a division of the national Society of Radiology.

Iceland

Currently, no formally competent paediatric radiologist is active in the country.

Norway

In Norway it was not until the early 1950s that paediatric radiology, as we know the subspeciality today, was established. For many years paediatrics, but in particular paediatric surgery, was almost exclusively centralized at the Rikshospitalet in Oslo. In 1950 a new Children's Hospital was inaugurated. S. Eek (Fig. 2), who had trained for several years with F. Ulfsparre at Crown Princess Louise Children's Hospital in Stockholm, became the first director. Eek was for a long time the radiologist mainly responsible for paediatric radiologic research work in Norway. His bibliography comprises 11 contributions published in international journals and one section in the book *Morbus Caeruleus* [5, 6]. Eek, who retired in 1975, had over the years, with great skill and experience, pursued the profession in training and inspiring young radiologists. One of them, G. Stake, President at the ESPR Meeting in Oslo, 1981, succeeded Eek as head of the department.

In 1966, K. Maurseth, who had spent several years with U. Rudhe in Stockholm, became associate chief radiologist in the department. In 1969 a position as paediatric radiologist was created at the University Hospital of Bergen (Haukeland Sygehus). S. Svendsen, who in 1972 moved to Kristiansand as head of a general radiology department, was succeeded by Maurseth.

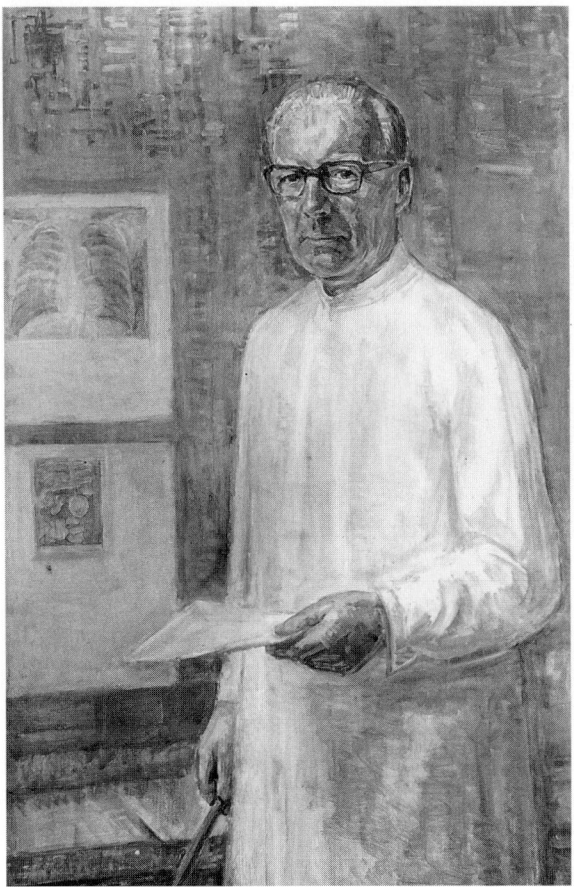

Figure 2
S. Eek, Norway

The paediatric radiology division of the Community Hospital of Oslo (Ullevål) was established in 1982, with T. Nordshus as radiologist in chief. At present there are no additional paediatric radiology divisions/departments in Norway.

Sweden

The first radiological examination in Sweden of a child with practical implications was performed on 1 April, 1898. A coin lodged in the upper oesophagus was identified and successfully removed. The original film was presented to Oscar II, King of Sweden, and was saved for the future in the Bernadotte Collection in Stockholm. However, the first roentgen equipment exclusively serving children's purposes was installed in 1907 in the Crown Princess Louise Children's Hospital (KLB) in Stockholm. The funds for the purchase were granted by the chairman of the board of directors. H. Waldenström, then a resident in the department of surgery, later professor of orthopaedic surgery at Karolinska Institutet, was among the first physicians responsible for the radiological examinations. Following a re-instalment of equipment in the 1920s, examinations were conducted by radiologists, among them E. Lysholm, later professor of diagnostic radiology (in particuar neuroradiology) at Karolinska Institutet. The panorama of disease was to a large extent that of tuberculous lesions.

However, paediatric radiological examinations also were carried out in the University Hospitals of Uppsala and Lund, in the Children's Hospital of Gothenburg, and in some County Hospitals. As early as 1927, Y. Olsson and G. Pallin of Kristianstad published a report concerning two cases of successful hydrostatic reduction of intussusception [15]. During the 1930s and 1940s great attention was paid to examination of acute abdominal disorders. The monograph [13] by Laurell of Uppsala set the pace as regards both technique and interpretation. The investigation by H. Hellmer of Lund concerning hydrostatic reduction of childhood intussusception [10] was effective in introducing the method in Scandinavia and elsewhere.

Specialized roentgen equipment, along with the advent of less toxic contrast media, contributed to improved diagnostics; this especially applied to congenital heart disease. In 1947, F. Ulfsparre, radiologist in chief at Crown Princess Louise Children's Hospital introduced angiocardiography into the routine; the following year no less than 70 examinations were performed. The collected experiences were accounted for in a book [19]. At about the same time the roentgen departments of the University Hospital in Lund and the Children's Hospital in Gothenburg brought the method into their routine programmes.

In 1954, L. Billing, then radiologist in the Orthopaedic Hospital of Gothenburg, made a lasting scientific contribution in presenting his investigation related to the proximal femur end in adolescents [2]. Four years later, L. Andrén and S. v. Rosen published a remarkable paper on the early diagnosis and treatment of CDH [1]. S. Scheller of Gothenburg contributed with a valuable study of the growth and ossification of the knee epiphyses [16].

The research work of S. R. Kjellberg (Fig. 3; radiologist in chief) and U. Rudhe (Fig. 4) in the newly erected Children's Hospital at Karolinska Sjukhuset meant an international breakthrough and global recognition of Swedish paediatric radiology. The volume on congenital heart disease [11] in 1954 and 1958 brought a wealth of new information from analysis of the results of a selective technique of angiocardiography as related to the physiology of cardiovascular abnormalities. An equally important and comprehensive work on the lower urinary tract was issued in 1957 [12].

When S. R. Kjellberg left the department in 1957 for a position as radiologist in chief in a new Department of Thoracic Radiology at Karolinska Sjukhuset, he was succeeded by U. Rudhe, who was in charge of the department until 1971. Numerous Swedish radiologists held, during a period of 20 years, more or less extensive terms of appointment for training in the paediatric radiology institution. In addition, quite a number of colleagues from overseas and various European countries stayed in the department. As a result of these visits, a considerable number of scientific publications are on record. Kjellberg and Rudhe later were elected full professors of general diagnostic radiology at Karolinska Institutet.

Following a 3-year residency in the department, O. Eklöf became associate radiologist in chief in 1965. He soon became deeply involved in teaching and research. In 1972 Eklöf succeeded Rudhe as head of the department. Eklöf retired in 1990.

In 1956, Kristina Ekengren became associate radiologist in chief at the Crown Princess Louise Children's Hospital. She succeeded Ulfsparre as head of the department in 1967. Three years later a new Children's Hospital was inaugurated in Stockholm (St. Göran). Ekengren remained in her position until her retirement in 1975. She was succeeded by W. Mortensson, who for more than 10 years had been in charge of paediatric radiology in Lund.

In the past, the City of Stockholm ran two additional Children's Hospitals, Sachska Barnsjukhuset and the Samaritan Children's Hospital. The radiological service in these hospitals during the 1940s was provided by general radiologists. In 1950, H. Gladnikoff became radiologist in chief of both units. A position as associate radiologist for the Samaritan Hospital was held by N. F. Bothén from 1960 until his retirement some 10 years later. Gladnikoff was succeeded by H. Ringertz in the mid 1970s. Ringertz was co-president of the IPR '91 and is to day full professor of general diagnostic radiology at Karolinska Sjukhuset.

Development of Paediatric Radiology in Scandinavia and Finland

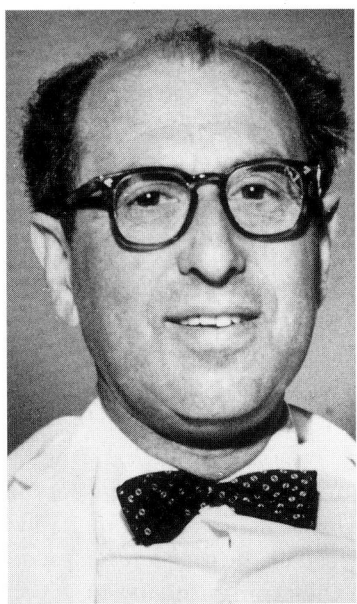

Figure 3
S. R. Kjellberg, Sweden

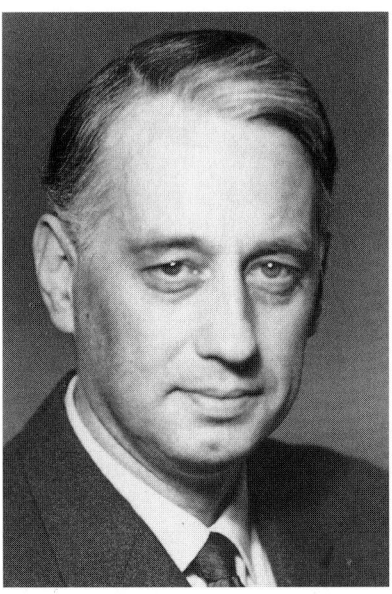

Figure 4
U. Rudhe, Sweden

H. Larsson was radiologist in chief in the Children's Hospital of Gothenburg from the late 1940s until his retirement in the mid 1970s. He was succeeded by B. Jacobsson as head of the department of radiology in the new Children's University Hospital of Gothenburg. Jacobsson left for other commitments in 1983, when I. Claesson succeeded him. Jacobsson is at present active again in the same department.

The University Hospitals in Malmö/Lund were for several years less specialized as regards paediatric radiology. From the early 1960s to 1983, G. Theander was director of the division of paediatric radiology in Malmö. H. Pettersson, now full professor of general diagnostic radiology in Lund, received his basic training in paediatric radiology with Theander. W. Mortensson held a similar position in Lund but moved to Stockholm in 1975. S. Laurin then took over as director of the division.

In Uppsala paediatric radiology was performed on a part-time basis by H. Lodin (later professor of general diagnostic radiology in Uppsala) and K. Bergström (later professor of neuroradiology in Uppsala) until H. Jorulf in 1976 was appointed head of the division for paediatric radiology. When Jorulf left because of other commitments in 1983, T. Lönnerholm took over. In 1990 Jorulf was appointed head of the division of paediatric radiology at Huddinge University Hospital.

C. Wegelius (later professor of general diagnostic radiology, University Hospital of Åbo/Turku) and J. Lind (later professor of paediatrics at Karolinska Sjukhuset) were involved in pioneer work related to cardiac and pulmonary abnormalities in the newborn [20].

Over the years, Swedish paediatric radiologists have published more than 800 papers, the vast majority of them in international journals. Considering the relatively few individuals involved, this achievement should be regarded as remarkable.

Swedish founding members of the ESPR were L. Andrén, S. Fagerberg, S. R. Kjellberg, S. Scheller and S. Welin. Currently, there are about 30 Swedish members of the Society. U. Rudhe was president at the Stockholm Meeting in 1965, O. Eklöf in 1976. H. Ringertz was co-president at the IPR '91 in Stockholm. The first postgraduate course in connection with ESPR meetings was arranged by Eklöf and Ringertz in 1976. Such courses, have been held at all subsequent meetings.

Ulf Rudhe was elected Honorary Member of the Society in 1976, O. Eklöf in 1987. Rudhe and Eklöf were created Honorary Members of the Society of Pediatric Radiology (SPR) in 1987, Ringertz in 1991.

In 1976 O. Eklöf and H. Ringertz were awarded the Alvarenga prize in appreciation of their article on a method of assessment of kidney size [7]. H. Ringertz and U. Erasmie received the Jacques Lefèbvre Memorial

Award in 1977 for their paper on appraisal of cranial suture width in neonates [8]. In recognition of Eklöf's contributions to paediatric radiology he received the C. Wegelius Medal and Award (1988).

Together with A. Crispin, K.-D. Ebel and A. Lassrich, Eklöf was instrumental in establishing the *Journal of Pediatric Radiology*. He was a member of the Editorial Board during the period 1973–1987.

The Swedish Society of Paediatric Radiology was founded in 1972. The majority of its approximately 50 members are active only part-time as paediatric radiologists. The Society is independent of the national Radiological Society.

Paediatric radiology was accepted as a subspeciality in 1975, becoming a speciality of its own in 1992. Training in paediatric radiology was established during the early 1950s. It was offered initially in the institutions in Stockholm. Later Gothenburg, Lund and Uppsala became involved in training programmes.

Currently, there are permanent positions for paediatric radiologists at four Stockholm hospitals, three of them being part of or affiliated with the Medical School. Corresponding positions are found in Malmö/Lund, Uppsala and Gothenburg. However, permanent positions for paediatric radiologists are lacking at the University Hospitals of Linköping and Umeå, and there are no such positions at other major community hospitals. Considering these facts, the number of residencies should be regarded as reasonable. However, adequate resources for obligatory short-term training of general radiologists do not exist.

The ESPR and its past meetings in Scandinavia, Finland and elsewhere have hardly affected the position of paediatric radiology in the Nordic countries. A full professorship in paediatric radiology has so far not been established.

References

1. Andrén L, von Rosen S (1958) The diagnosis of dislocation of the hip in newborns and primary result of immediate treatment. Acta Radiol 49:89–95
2. Billing L (1954) Roentgen examination of the proximal femur end in children and adolescents. Acta Radiol Suppl 110
3. Brünner S (1964) Cystis pulm. A clinical-radiological study. Munksgaard, Copenhagen
4. Brünner S (1964) Radiological examination of temporal bone in infants and children. Radiology 82:401–406
5. Eek S (1949) Roentgenological examination of morbus caeruleus. In: Mannheimer E (ed) Morbus caeruleus. An analysis of 114 cases of congenital heart disease with cyanosis. Karger, Basel

6. Eek S, Knutrud O (1962) Megacolon congenitum Hirschsprung. A follow-up study of 63 patients. J Oslo City Hosp 12:245–270
7. Eklöf O, Ringertz H (1976) Kidney size in children. A method of assessment. Acta Radiol 17:617–625
8. Erasmie U, Ringertz H (1976) The width of cranial sutures in the neonate. An objective method of assessment. Acta Radiol 17:565–572
9. Heikel P-E (1967) Postmortal changes in the lung. A roentgenographic and bacteriological follow-up study on a pediatric series and on animals with experimental pneumonia. Acta Radiol Suppl 264
10. Hellmer H (1947) Intussusception in children. Diagnosis and therapy with barium enema. Acta Radiol Suppl 65
11. Kjellberg SR, Mannheimer E, Rudhe U, Jonsson B (1954) Diagnosis of congenital heart disease. Year Book Publishers, Chicago
12. Kjellberg SR, Ericsson NO, Rudhe U (1957) The lower urinary tract in childhood. Almqvist and Wiksell, Stockholm
13. Laurell H (1939) Om Röntgen vid Akuta Bukfall (Swedish). Almqvist and Wiksell, Uppsala
14. Nordentorft JM (1943) Value of barium enema in diagnosis and treatment of intussusception in children. Illustrated by about 500 Danish cases. Acta Radiol Suppl 51
15. Olsson Y, Pallin G (1927) Über das Bild der akuten Darminvagination bei Röntgenuntersuchung und über Desinvagination mit Hilfe von Kontrastlavements. Acta Chir Scand 61:371–383
16. Scheller S (1965) Roentgenographic studies on epiphyseal growth and ossification of the knee. Acta Radiol Suppl 195
17. Stenström R (1967) Arthrography of the knee joint in children. A classification and results of conservative treatment. Acta Radiol Suppl 281
18. Thomsen G (1955) Hiatus hernia in children. Acta Radiol Suppl 129
19. Ulfsparre F (1949) Angiocardiography in morbus caeruleus. In: Mannheimer E (ed) Morbus caeruleus. An analysis of 114 cases of congenital heart disease with cyanosis. Karger, Basel
20. Wegelius C, Lind J (1953) The role of the exposure rate in angiocardiography. Acta Radiol 39:177–191

Development of Pediatric Radiology in Austria

W. Swoboda

Austria is one of the countries of Europe where pediatric radiology is still not acknowledged as an official medical subspeciality with a standard curriculum for radiologists and/or pediatricians. While before and after World War II radiodiagnostic procedures in the major children's hospitals were usually performed by pediatricians interested in and somewhat trained in X-ray diagnostics, this changed in the 1970s and 1980s, together with the introduction of new and more sophisticated imaging technologies. At the three University Children's Hospitals (Graz, Innsbruck, and Vienna) full-time positions for doctors with complete specialization in radiology together with extensive experience in pediatric radiology do exist. Moreover, three persons (Drs. Gassner, Weiss, and Vergesslich) completed the full curriculum for specialization in pediatrics as well as radiodiagnostics, which means a total of 12 years of postgraduate training!

In most of the nonacademic Children's Hospitals throughout the country there are radiologists with special training in pediatric problems in full- or part-time positions. The pediatric departments of the large general hospitals usually still lack such specialists, and physicians with experience in pediatric radiology continue to bridge that gap.

In the official curriculum for specialization in radiology, a training of 3–6 months at an acknowledged institution for pediatric radiology, primarily university departments, is strongly recommended. Though not (yet) compulsory, it will be included in the new radiology training program in the not too distant future.

Historically, for many years Austrian pediatricians have contributed significantly to the field of pediatric radiology. To be mentioned are the studies of H. C. Wimberger on rickets, scurvy and congenital syphilis in the young child (1925), as well as the work of R. Priesel on tuberculosis (1930). Engelmann's disease refers to the Austrian radiologist G. Engelmann, who described this entity for the first time in 1929. Interestingly, this "tradition" of studying development and diseases of the skeletal system in childhood continued later with numerous publications and two books by W. Swoboda. His close co-worker at the Vienna University Children's Hospital was H.G. Wolf, also a pediatrician. Wolf was primarily interested in radiological imaging of the gastrointestinal system of children, following his excellent basic training at A. Lassrich's institute in Hamburg. He also inaugurated a monthly session with very informal but highly successful discussions on unusual or unexplained observations related to pediatric radiology. This institution was carried on after the early and tragic death of Dr. Wolf in 1976, and it attracts participants from many different medical disciplines even today.

At the beginning of the ESPR, W. Swoboda (Vienna) and H. Wendler (Graz) were the representatives from Austria, soon joined by G. Felsenreich and H.G. Wolf (both Vienna), all four pediatricians. The rapid development of radiology and related techniques in the past two decades has also profoundly changed this list of names. To date, the following persons are active (or associate) members of the ESPR: Richard Fotter (Ass.), Ingmar Gassner (Ass.), Walter Ponhold (Ass.), Gertraud Puschnik-Maurer (Act.), and Klara Vergesslich (Act.).

The History of Pediatric Radiology in Czechoslovakia

S. Tůma, E. Kolihová and A. Rubín

In 1897, a carpenter who had swallowed an unusually long nail, was brought to Prague Surgical Clinic of Professor Eiselt. A young medical assistant was on duty at the time, Rudolf Jedlička, an enthusiast of new methods, and he took the patient to a pub called "The Black Horse" located in Na Příkopech street. The owner, Mr. Cífka, had installed for the pleasure of his guests the first X-ray apparatus in what was later to become Czechoslovakia. The X-ray picture, obtained after a very long exposition on January 12, 1897, showed the unusual position of the swallowed nail, and the nail was then removed by the surgeons (Tošovský 1990).

This was the first intervention performed in our country on the basis of an X-ray examination. Rudolf Jedlička, who later became Professor of Surgery and Orthopedics at the Czech Medical Faculty of Charles University in Prague, dedicated himself to radiology. He was the first to publish X-ray findings on children's diseases in Bohemia. On November 14, 1898, he demonstrated to the Association of Czech Physicians and published in the *Journal of Czech Physicians* observations of X-ray findings in children: a fracture of the right radius in an 11-year-old boy after a fall, a needle located in the palm of a 10-year-old girl, and a shotgun wound of the left shoulder in a 14-year-old girl, as well as a pleural exsudate in pulmonary metastasis of a femoral osteosarcoma in a girl of 15 years (Jedlička 1899). He devoted himself throughout his life as a surgeon to the application of radiology. In the end, he had to pay for his enthusiasm; he, an esteemed surgeon, had to undergo amputation of three fingers of his left hand due to post-radiation changes.

At that time, Béla Alexander, a native of the town of Kežmarok in Slovakia, was the first professor of radiology. He worked in Budapest, and attempted to obtain plastic pictures (Alexander 1906).

At the German Medical Faculty of Charles University in Prague, Basch directed his interest to the diagnosis of chest organs and described the appearance of the thymus in children (Basch 1903). This work was continued by Fischl, who became Professor of Pediatrics, and later by B. Epstein.

At the end of the 1920s, Švejcar in Bratislava performed the first bronchography in children, as well as the first excretory urography. He worked together with an excellent radiologist, Dreuschuh. In 1930 and 1931 after the return from Bratislava, when the era of both professors of paediatrics, Brdlík and Švejcar, in Prague was beginning, the first X-ray apparatus was installed in the Czech Pediatric Clinic in Prague. It was of novel design, especially equipped for the examination of infants. It was designed by the Czech engineer Vinopal, later owner of the Meta Company. Vinopal produced this apparatus exclusively for the Pediatric Clinic, and he installed it on credit; it was paid for later by the Czechoslovak Red Cross. In this way he outdid his competitors, the firms Siemens and Koch und Sterzl.

In the "Nalezinec", the foundling hospital in Prague, Dr. Žahourek worked as a radiologist (Švejcar 1987). Individual observations of bone and other diseases in children were described by Šváb (Šváb 1927) and others. In 1933 Hečko and Vychytil detected congenital heart diseases by means of X-ray. Their description of a narrow vascular peduncle in the cardiac silhouette of the transposition of the great arteries is the first explanation of the diagnostic features of this disease (Hečko and Vychytil 1933). Dr. V. Volfová studied and more clearly described the X-ray findings in congenital heart disease (Volfová 1944). Prusík and Volicer attempted to examine peripheral arteries (Prusík and Volicer 1928). Following the work of Moniz in 1930, there were a number of authors (Hněvkovský 1932, 1934; Kňažovický 1933; Matulay and Kauzál 1934) who attempted to perform arteriography.

During the war and postwar years the evolution of this method continued. Articles were published mostly in *Časopis lékařů českých*, founded in 1862. *Acta radiologica et cancerologica bohemoslovenica* was edited by Šváb and Škorpil from 1946. *Československá radiologie* was started in 1955 by Professor Jaromír Kolář. Today it is the official journal of the Czech and Slovak societies of radiology (Věšín 1989).

In 1950, Padovcová, Horák, and Bor published a paper on angiocardiography in children. At that time their work was unique – the first "sui generis" in central Europe. In February 1949, Dr. Hana Padovcová had started performing angiocardiography in children with congenital heart disease. She was assisted by several radiologists of that time, Bedřich Horák and Antonín Rubín, as well as by cardiologist Imrich Bor. The examinations were performed by manual injection of contrast agent into a peripheral vein – most frequently the jugular vein. Under fluoroscopic control on a standard fluoroscopic table with manual exchange of cassettes, this medical team, assisted by two X-ray technicians and one nurse, managed to record the flow of contrast agent through the heart and pulmonary circulation as well as the outflow into the systemic circulation, on a set of six (!) pictures. We present one of the first documents, made in April 1949 (Fig. 1).

After World War II, the Department of Radiology of the Pediatric University Hospital in Prague served Pediatric Clinics I and II, under Professor Josef Švejcar (at present the nestor of world pediatrics) and Professor Jiří Brdlík. A large amount of scientific clinical and X-ray material was accumulated there. The first head of this department was Jaroslav Sommer, followed by Bedřich Horák, Antonín Rubín, and Oldřich Šnobl. Pediatric surgery was developed by Miroslav Hladík. In 1953, A. Rubín and O. Šnobl published the basic lecture notes for medical students, i.e., the ground work for the field of pediatric radiology in this country (Rubín and Šnobl 1953). At that time, Josef Houštěk, later the successor to Professor Brdlík, and Dean of the Faculty of Pediatrics from 1953 when it was established, dedicated himself to X-ray diagnostics in children. The trio of authors – J. Houštěk, A. Rubín and O. Šnobl – later published a monograph entitled "X-ray Diagnosis of Bony Alterations in Diseases of the Pediatric Age" (Houštěk et al. 1958).

A. Rubín (Fig. 2), later Professor of Pediatrics, laid the foundation for the concept of pediatric radiology, correlating X-ray findings with their clinical basis. Later he extended his activities as a pediatrician to the adolescent age-group. Some of his further research was devoted to X-ray problems. He participated in the promotion of Czechoslovak pediatric radiology on the international level. He was a long-term member of the Editorial Council of *Pediatric Radiology*, vice-president and, in 1982, president to the ESPR, in charge of the 19th Congress of our Society in Prague. He was assisted by the secretaries, Jiří Vymlátil and Stanislav Tůma. He published numerous articles on disorders of bone and the alimentary tract in children and of the urinary tract in children and adolescents (Rubín 1967; Rubín et al. 1976; Rubín and Pospíšil 1956).

O. Šnobl (Fig. 3) extended our understanding of X-ray changes with special attention to the lungs and the mediastinum, particularly in his publications on diaphragmatic hernias in children and the differential diagnosis of pulmonary sequestrations (Šnobl 1956). Together with Miroslav Hladík, they wrote a basic and – for the time being – the only textbook of pediatric radiology in our language (Hladík and Šnobl 1963). In 1981, with Václav Mydlil he published a monograph entitled "Radiodiagnosis of Respiratory Organs and the Alimentary Tract in Newborns". As lecturer in radiology in the Pediatric Faculty of Charles University in Prague, Snobl educated a whole generation of pediatricians graduating from this faculty. Furthermore, he initiated a postgraduate training program for radiologists

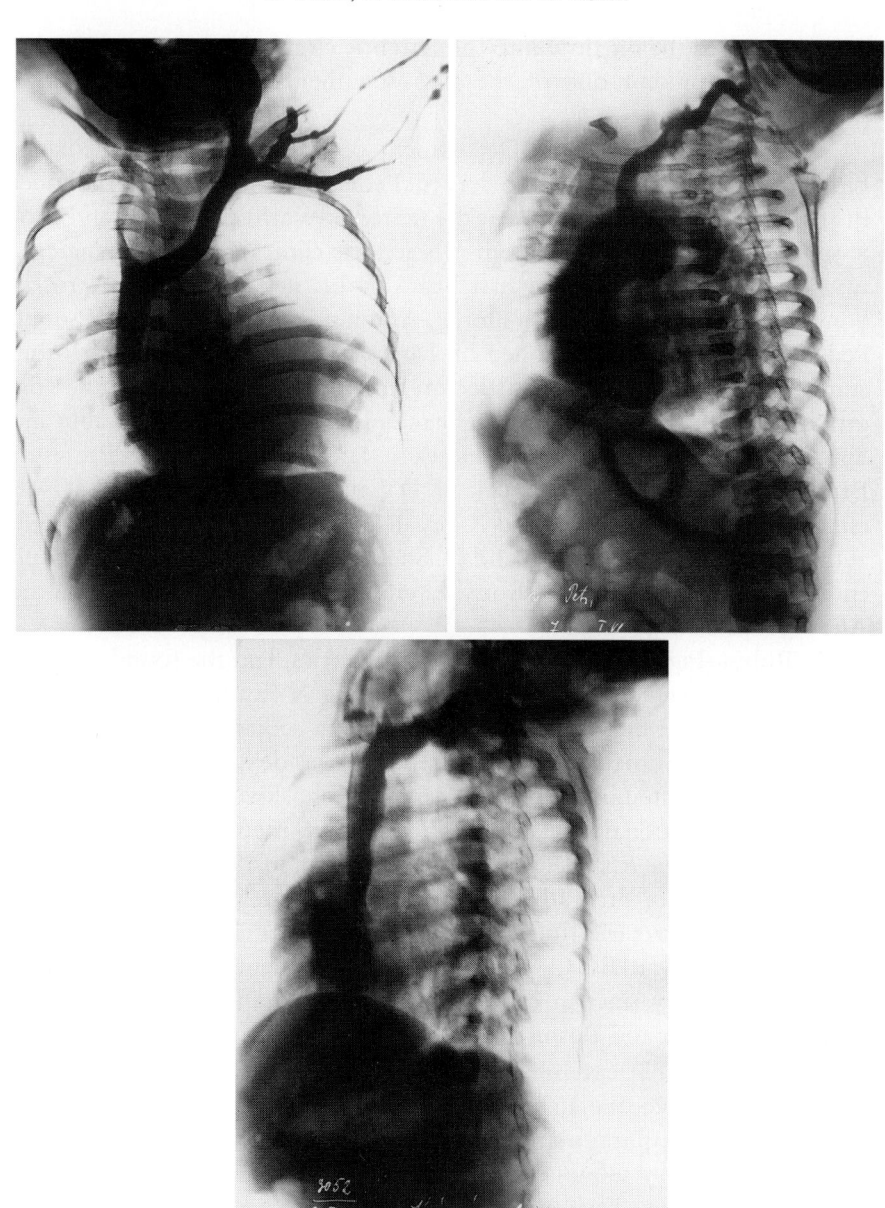

Figure 1
X-rays made in April 1949 to record the flow of contrast agent

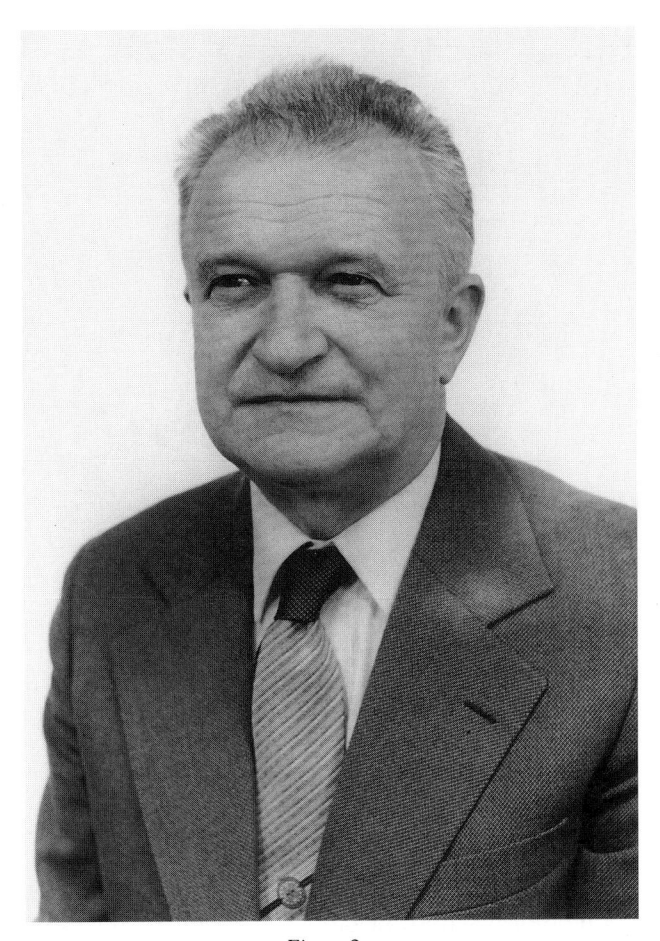

Figure 2
Antonín Rubín, professor of pediatrics and President of the ESPR in 1982, who organized the 19th congress, held in Prague

in pediatric problems. The Czechoslovak Society of Pediatric Radiology is the result of all these activities.

In 1962 a Central Radiodiagnostic Section in the Pediatric University Hospital in Prague was created, with Eva Kolihová (Fig. 4) as its head. In this unit, new personalities such as Jiří Abraham, Hedvika Bělíková, Jaromír Hořák, Dagmar Obenbergerová, Štefan Ridzoň, Stanislav Tůma, and Marie Zítková successively were trained. They continue to further develop the field of pediatric radiology. With the opening of the Pediatric Hospital in Motol, in 1967, a new era, the so-called Motol era of the Prague

S. Tůma, E. Kolihová and A. Rubín

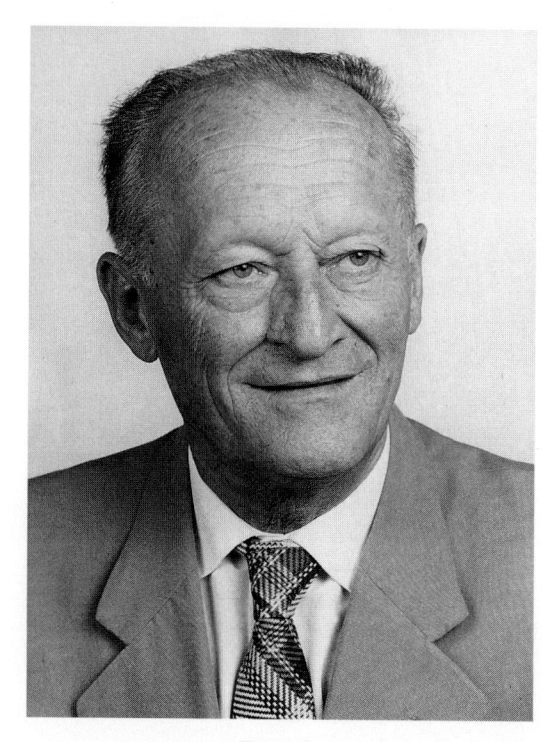

Figure 3
Oldřich Šnobl, professor of pediatrics

Pediatric Radiological school began. The Head of this department, Eva Kolihová, developed it by virtue of her personality. She was an allround knowledgeable pediatric radiologist and she trained many future specialists in this field (Kolihová and Obenbergerová 1983). She started to examine pediatric-oncologic patients with angiography and ultrasound (Kolihová et al. 1984). She is the author of instructional films and teaching texts for students of the former Pediatric Faculty – now the Second Medical Faculty of Charles University in Prague in the University Hospital Motol.

At the Cardiology Center of the University Hospital Motol, Stanislav Tůma (Fig. 5) devoted himself to angiography and to the development of interventional methods in the vascular system in children (Tůma et al. 1991). Since 1990, he has been the head of the X-ray department. It's name was changed in November 1991 to "Clinic for Imaging Methods" of the University Hospital at Motol, serving as a teaching center for the Second Medical Faculty of Charles University in Prague.

The History of Pediatric Radiology in Czechoslovakia

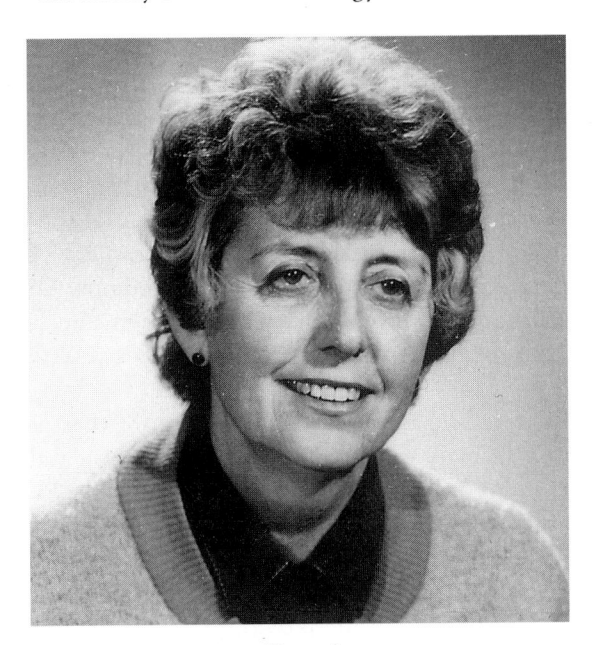

Figure 4
Eva Kolihová

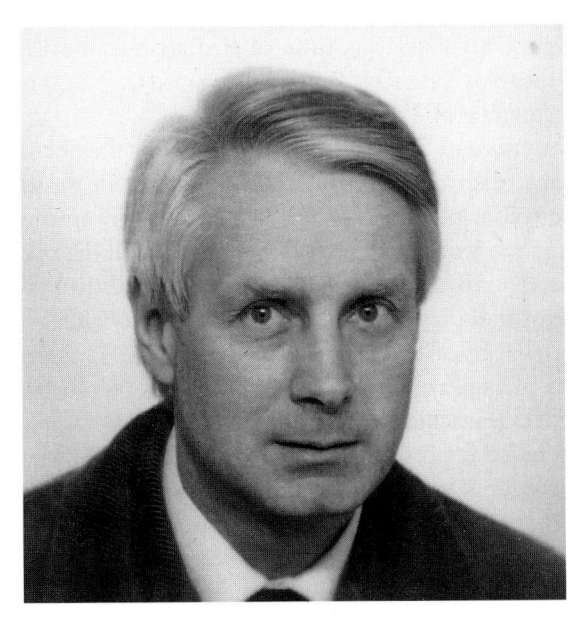

Figure 5
Stanislav Tůma

Until World War II, separate pediatric beds were available only in Pediatric Clinics in Prague, Brno, and Bratislava. At the beginning of May 1939, a Pediatric Department was constituted also in the Regional Hospital in Olomouc, founded in 1896. The head physician at that time became Dr. Antonín Mores. A further pediatric department was established at Frýdek. The department in Olomouc was enlarged after the war, and with the founding of Palacký University in 1946 it became a clinic. Pediatric problems were treated by the radiologists Dr. Huf and now Dr. Michálková. The first successful operation of a ductus arteriosus in Czechoslovakia was performed in this pediatric department in 1948 by Professor Rapant (Navrátil 1980).

In the Czech republic there are presently more than 70 radiologists working either exclusively or predominantly as pediatric radiologists. The Prague Motol center employs 12 pediatric radiologists. In Prague there are independent diagnostic units of pediatric radiology at the Children's University Hospital (with Lejská and Jakubcová), at Krč (Urbanová and Kocourková), in the Children's University Hospital at Vinohrady (Václav Brychnáč), and at Bulovka (Černušáková). Independent pediatric radiologists work also in larger hospitals in Bohemia — Eliška Chramostová in České Budějovice, Eva Valentová in the University Hospital Plzeň, and Adolf Kopecký in the University Hospital in Hradec Králové. In the University Hospital in Brno (Moravia) the teaching institution for pediatrics of today's Masaryk University, a Clinic of Pediatric Radiodiagnosis was established; the head is Jaroslav Procházka, who is also president of the Czechoslovak Society of Pediatric Radiology.

The representative of Slovakian Radiology after the Second World War was an excellent diagnostician and radiotherapist, Professor Lanyi, who was also interested in pediatric problems. He was an eminent personality and specialized in osteology. Classical pediatric radiodiagnosis was represented by Prunyi in Bratislava. At present this tradition is continued by Macek in the Hospital Na Kramároch and by his associate, Stanová. Professor Démant in charge of the Pediatric Clinic of the University of Košice, was specialized in nephrology. In this clinic Julis Veréb became the first Doctor of Sciences (Habilitation) among pediatric radiologists in Czechoslovakia. At present he is president of the Slovakian Radiological Society.

Pediatric problems were also treated by a whole range of radiologists, not specialized in pediatric radiology. In the first place should be mentioned Professor J. Kolář, the present president of the Czech Radiological Society, J. Beran and H. Zídková, who devoted their attention to osteology. They published a wide range of observations on disorders of the pediatric age group.

References

Alexander B (1906) Erzeugung plastischer Röntgenbilder. Fortschr Röntgenstr 1:46
Basch (1903) Über Ausschaltung der Thymusdrüse. Wien Med Wschr 31
Hečko I, Vychytil D (1933) Klinická a rentgenologická diagnostika transpozice velkých cév srdečních. Čas Lék čes 72:676–681
Hladík M, Šnobl O (1963) Pediatrická rentgenologie. St zdrav nakl, Prague
Hněvkovský O (1932) Arteriografie končetin a mozku. Čas Lék čes 599
Houštěk J, Rubín A, Šnobl O (1956) Rentgenový obraz kostních změn při některých onemocněních dětského věku. St zdrav nakl, Prague
Jedlička R (1899) O skiagrafii a skiaskopii paprsky Röntgenovými a jejich diagnostické ceně v chirurgii. Čas Lék čes 1–14
Kňazovický J (1933) O arteriografiích. Čas Lék čes 353
Matulay K, Kauzál G (1934) O mozgovej arteriografii. Bratisl Lek Listy 24
Kolihová E, Obenbergerová D (1983) Intestinal obstruction during the first days of life. Ann Radiol 26:161–167
Kolihová E, Zítková M, Šuchmová M, Jirásek M, Weinreb M (1984) Nesnáze v radiodiagnostice dětských nádorů. Prakt Lékař 64:15–16
Navrátil M (1990) Padesát let nemocniční pediatrie v Olomouci. Čs Pediat 45:244–246
Padovcová H, Horák B, Bor I (1950) Angiokardiografie u vrozených malformací srdce. Čas Lék čes 89:217–225
Prusík B, Volicer L (1928) Rentgenografické vyšetřování cév periferních (arteriografie). Čas Lék čes 41
Prusík B, Volicer L (1928) Klinické výsledky rtg-grafie arterií po vstříknutí jodového oleje. Čas Lék čes 498–683
Rubín A (1967) Ileus und ileusartige Zustände im frühen Kindesalter. Thieme, Stuttgart
Rubín A, Biganovská V, Blažek T (1976) Urinary tract disease in adolescence. A radiological and clinical view. Pediat Radiol 5:254
Rubín A, Pospíšil V (1956) Tvar a velikost tureckého sedla u dětského diabetu. Čs Pediat 8:63
Rubín A, Šnobl O (1953) Některé kapitoly z dětské rentgenologie. St ped nakl, Prague
Šváb V (1927) Příspěvek ke vrozeným tvarovým a segmentačním úchylkám páteře. Roč Čsl Spol Rentgenol Radiol, Prague, pp 43–47
Švejcar J (1987) Česká dětská klinika v pražském nalezinci v mé paměti i v životě. Čs Pediat 42:351–358, 429–435
Šnobl O (1965) Die angeborenen Zwerchfellhernien. Acta Univ Carol, Prague
Šnobl O, Mydlil V (1981) Radiodiagnostika pneumopatií novorozeneckého a kojeneckého věku. Avicenum, Prague
Tošovský VV (1990) Padesát let chirurgem. Univ Karlova, Prague, pp 170–171
Tůma S, Povýšilová V, Škovránek J, Tax P (1991) Klinická morfologie defektu komorového septa. Čs Pediat 46:2–6
Tůma S, Šamánek M, Tax P, Hučín B (1991) Zur Frage der transvasalen Katheterembolisation von Kollateralarterien bei der Pulmonalatresie. Radiol Diagn 32:176–180
Tůma S, Špatenka J, Tax P, Honěk T, Kostelka M, Horák D (1991) Intervenční embolisační léčba angiodysplázií u dětí. Čs Radiol 45:1–7
Věšín S (1989) Vývoj a výhledy naší rentgenologie. Čs Radiol 43:133–138
Volfová V (1944) Vrozená vada srdeční se zvláštním roentgenovým obrazem. Čas Lék čes 83:370

The History of Paediatric Radiology in Germany

E. WILLICH and K.-D. EBEL

The Early Era – from 1895 to 1962

By 1896, the year after the discovery of X-rays, 21 reports had already been published on their application in children. At that time Germany was one of the world's leading countries in medicine, and by April 1896, a paediatrician in Munich, von Ranke, had reported on the ossification of the wrist in children. In July, Angerer, also in Munich, demonstrated rachitic changes. In Graz, Austria, Escherich was able to install X-ray equipment. In those days an X-ray exposure of the wrist took 10 min and so younger children had to be anaesthetized (chloroform). The Charité children's clinic in Berlin under Heubner received its first X-ray laboratory in 1903. In 1912, also in Berlin, Reyher published the first German monograph: the skeleton alone covered 150 pages, all other organs only 19 pages. X-ray examination was used mainly in rickets, skeletal lues, malformations, and systemic skeletal diseases, after 1908 also for tuberculosis. Hamburger published a monograph on tuberculosis in 1912 and by 1923 three such books had appeared.

In those days paediatrics was hardly referred to in the major radiology books (Goett in Rieder and Rosenthal 1913). After 1920 some important books on paediatric radiology were published by Duken (1924), Saupe (1925, 1929), and Gralka (1927). The problem of how to obtain adequate X-rays and how to avoid repeat exposures resulted in a preoccupation with fixation devices. The inventor of the first "infant chair" at the turn of the century remains unknown. In 1908 Großer described such a device. The support bench was introduced by Wimberger in 1922, to which a Glisson's sling (Fig. 1) was added 4 years later by Viethen. In 1934 the device was further modified with movable metal rods. Lutz Schall (1894–1978) was the pioneer of German paediatric radiology (see "Bremen" and "Tübingen"). For decades Schall, honorary member of the ESPR, devoted his efforts to the problem of immobilizing babies for X-ray examination. In 1928 he constructed the "Schall's bench" – a designation to which he

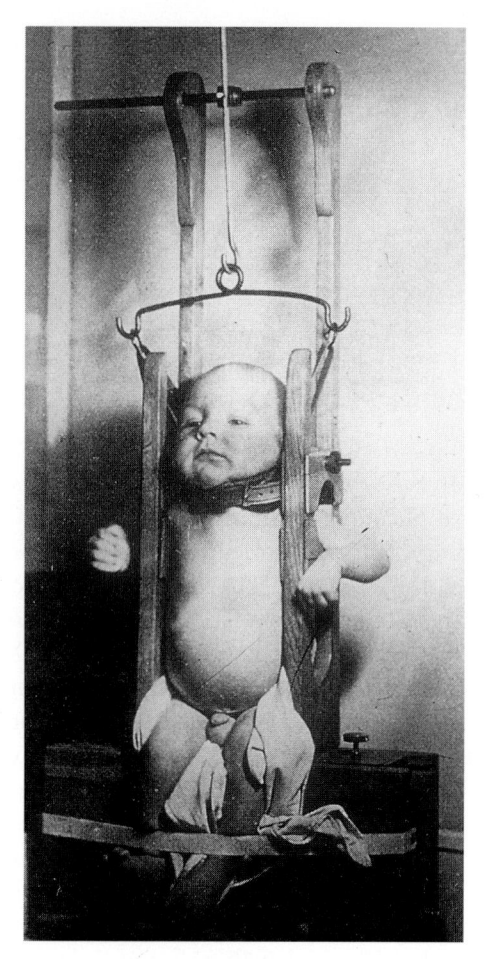

Figure 1
Modification of the support bench of Wimberger as described by Viethen in 1926, also introducing Glisson's sling

protested in vain. Its basic principle was a supporting system that used the individual weight of the body (Figs. 2, 3). His main intent was to reduce the amount of radiation applied by avoiding repeat exposures and also to have a helping person support the patients. In 1962 he introduced the "Paidoskop" as an attachment to the generally available X-ray machines, allowing positional changes of the child during fluoroscopy (Fig. 4), and specialized paediatric X-ray machines – pediatrix (CGR/Paris, France) and

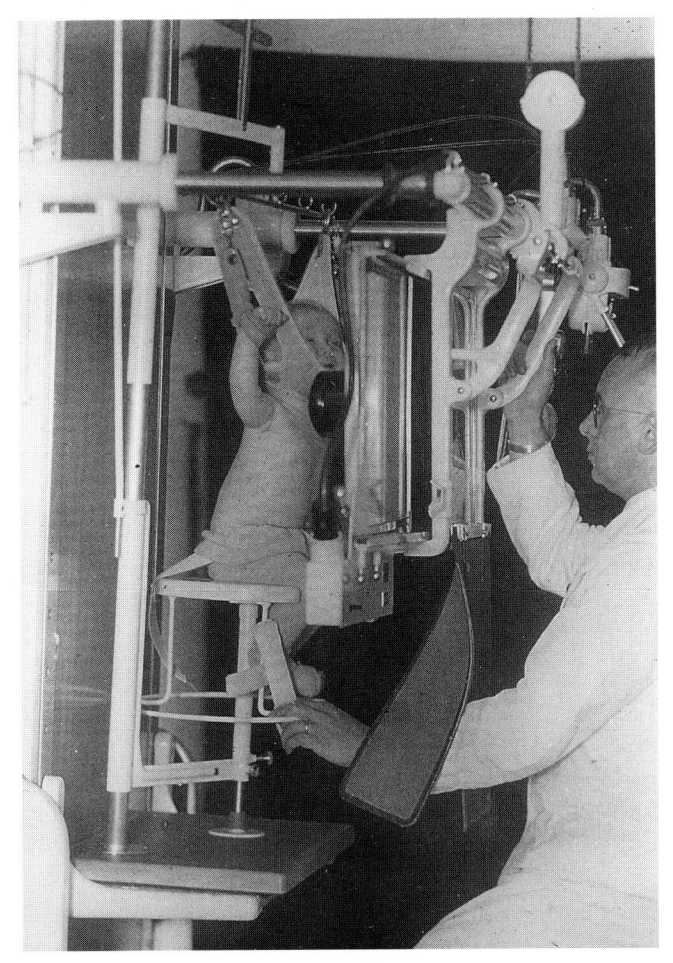

Figure 2
Support system using the principle of a nonconnecting support system – "Schall's bench" – 1928. On the *right*: Lutz Schall

"infantoscop" (Siemens, Erlangen, Germany) were the final result. In 1950 the cellophane wrap ("Babix") which is still widely used today, especially for chest films, was introduced.

During World War II, there was complete stagnation and it was not until around 1950 that some paediatricians devoted their work to radiology. The result was the simultaneous appearance of two standard books by M. A. Lassrich and F. Schmidt together with Weber in 1955.

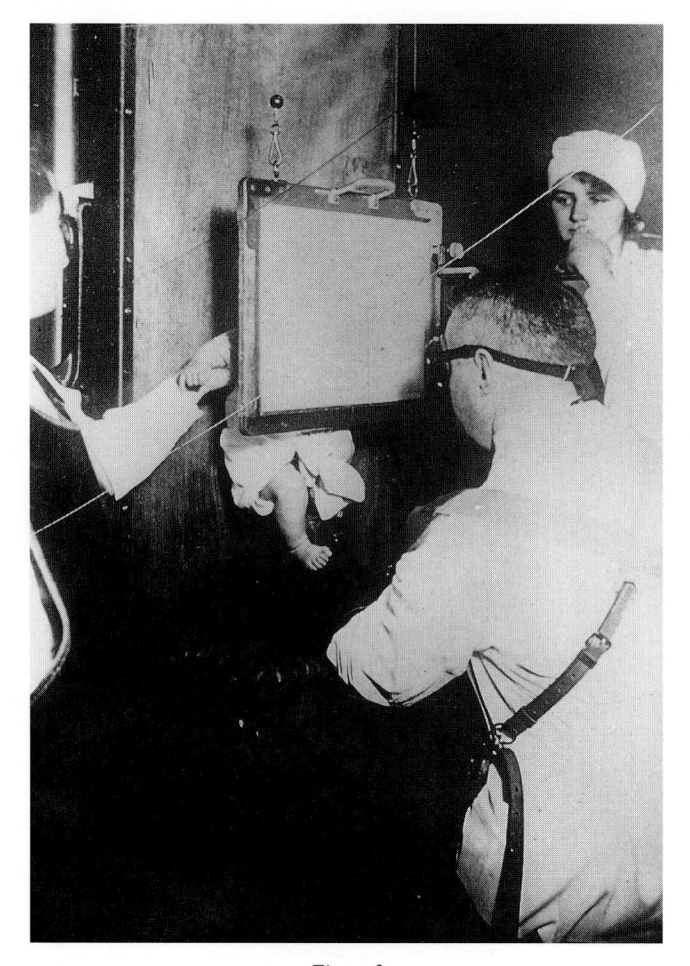

Figure 3
Roentgen investigation according to Grävinghoff 1932: two nurses are supporting the child, investigator: Lutz Schall

Paediatric Radiology in Germany Since 1963

The initial impetus to form an organisation of German-speaking paediatric radiologists came at the first Paris meeting in 1963. Ten participants from Germany were present there, and at the first ESPR meeting in Paris in 1964 already twice as many. On 17 September 1963, on the occasion of a

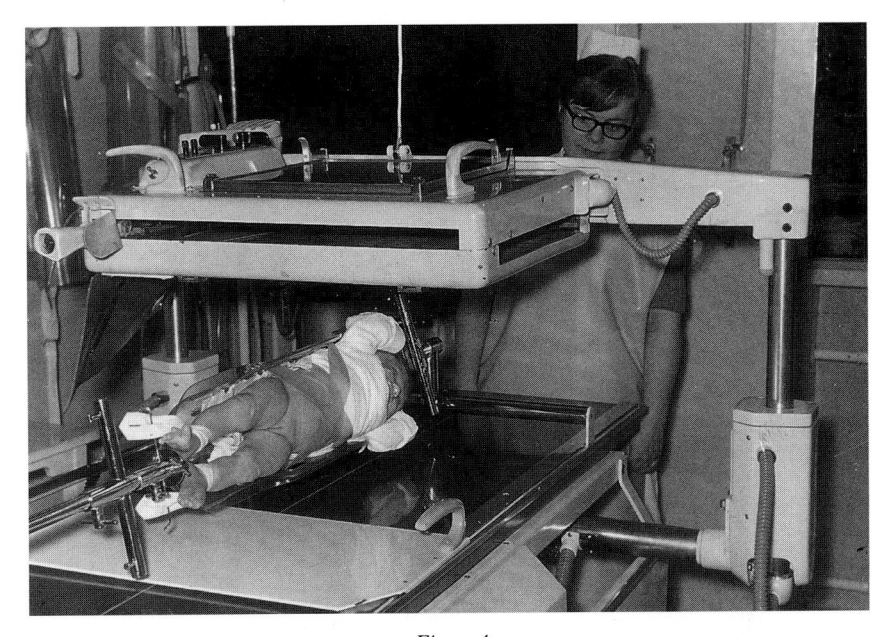

Figure 4
Paidoskop with a motor driven manipulation system of the restrained child during an investigation in supine position. Construction according to Lutz Schall (1962)

paediatric meeting in Cologne, Germany, the foundation for a "working group – paediatric radiology" was laid, with M. A. Lassrich in charge. During subsequent years this group always met in connection with the annual meeting of the paediatricians. In 1965 in Nuremberg, Germany, paediatric radiology was the main topic at the meeting of the German Radiological Society for the first time. At that time, there were only 11 full-time paediatric radiologists. A countercurrent was unsuccessful, having tried to emphasize the paediatric orientation. By 1968 at a meeting in Bonn, 48 members voted to an "official society". At that time it was also decided to start an international, English-language journal. M. A. Lassrich had been particularly active in the preparation and an editorial board of 29 paediatric radiologists from all corners of the world gave their support to seven editors and three specialists as advisory board. Thus *Pediatric Radiology* was born, published by Springer in 1973. Over the past 20 years, the number of copies printed has reached 1200.

At the independently organized annual meeting in 1969 the members decided to become more closely affiliated with the German Radiological Society by forming a section of that body. In 1970 the name was changed

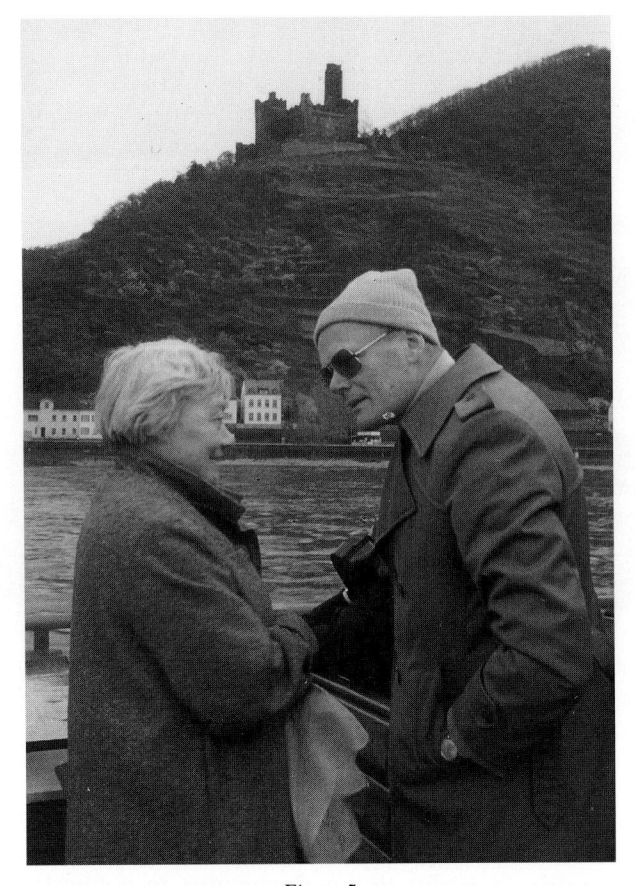

Figure 5
"East meets West" at the ESPR Congress Cologne in 1979. Boat trip on the Rhine river after the congress. (Prof. Baklanowa from Moscow and K. D. Ebel)

to "*Gesellschaft für Pädiatrische Radiologie – GPR*" (Paediatric Radiology Society). Its purpose was to provide a forum for all German-speaking paediatric radiologists.

Its first board consisted of M. A. Lassrich, H. J. Kaufmann, W. Schuster, I. Greinacher and as its most active secretary K.-D. Ebel. The membership had grown to 84. In 1971 F. Heuck, a general radiologist, suggested for the first time openly that paediatric radiology be recognised as a subspeciality. In response the paediatricians indicated that X-ray diagnosis was part and parcel of the catalogue of topics to be taught to future paediatricians and therefore paediatric radiology should be an integral part of paediatrics.

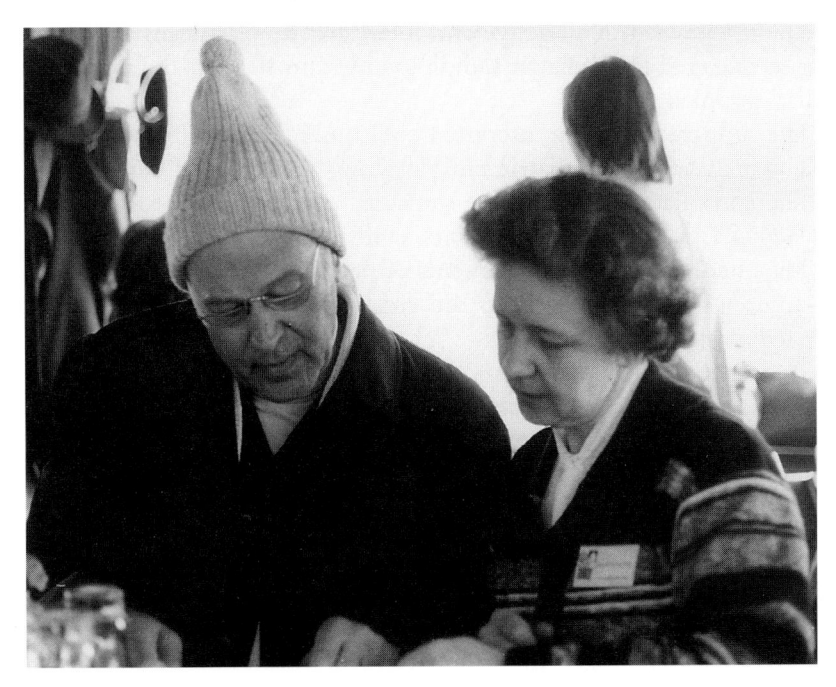

Figure 6
Same occasion as in Figure 5. The most frequent visitor from Russia, N. Konstantinowa from Moscow and E. Willich

E. Willich was elected as chairman of the GPR in 1972. His aims were:

1. To attain recognition of paediatric radiology as a subspeciality of radiology. This was discussed at the business meeting of the German Medical Society in1978 but was tabled by the paediatricians.
2. The opening-up of the society for German-speaking paediatric radiologists, in particular from the then Eastern European countries. With the help of K. Gefferth (see Fig. 2 in the chapter on Hungary), paediatric radiologists from the East, first from Hungary and then from Poland and Czechoslovakia as well, participated. In some instances fellowships could be arranged. Our colleagues from the former German Democratic Republic (GDR) found it extremely difficult to come to our meetings, particularly when held in West Germany. Thus it was particularly good that we could hold GPR meeting in Switzerland, Austria and Holland. During a trip to the Soviet Union contacts were established, and in 1979 a Soviet delegation participated in the ESPR Congress in Cologne (Figs. 5, 6).

3. The integration of all active and interested paediatricians and radiologists engaged in paediatric radiology. Within 10 years the membership had doubled to 240.
4. The support of young interested colleagues through fellowships.
5. The inclusion of paediatric radiology in the society of radiologists.
6. The compilation of objective statistical data as a basis for employing paediatric radiology departmental staff.
7. The establishment of departments of paediatric radiology in the larger children's hospitals and also the creation of permanent positions for paediatric radiologists.
8. To improve interdisciplinary cooperation with paediatric oncology, gastroenterology, orthopaedics and others.

When the new chairman, W. Schuster, took over in 1982, there were 18 paediatric radiologists in independent positions and 37 simply employed, all of them in hospitals. In Karlsruhe at the 1987 meeting of the delegates of the German Physicians, paediatric radiology was finally recognised as a radiologic subspeciality. A scientific prize was set up for the best paper presented at the annual meeting. Committees were formed within the GPR for professional and scientific problems. The integration of the paediatric radiologists from the former GDR as a result of the unification of Germany was an important task after 1990. When W. Schuster was replaced by M. Reither in November 1992 as chairman, the membership of GPR consisted of 290 members from 13 European countries. There are seven honorary members, whereas in the ESPR six honorary members are from Germany.

Paediatric Radiology
in the Former German Democratic Republic

A section of the Society for Medical Radiology of the GDR was founded in 1966 by H. Buttenberg (died in 1972). In 1971 this group joined with a similarly named section within the paediatric society. From then until 1990, there were two meetings annually, one independently and the other alternating with the annual meeting of the paediatricians and the radiologists. Good regular contact existed among the specialities. From 1973 on, H. J. Preuss was in charge, assisted by I. Nitz, F. Erfurt, G. Berger, J. Friedrich and E. Rupprecht. In 1980 D. Hörmann followed as chairman. Subsequently, on a 2-year basis, instructional courses were organised by the Academy for continuing Medical Education. The last chairwoman (1987—

1990) was Helga Wiersbitzky. At that time the highest membership was reached – 56 paediatric radiologists, 21 of them women. Two participants from the GDR were officially allowed to participate in the Third ESPR Congress in 1965. Subsequently, one or two members could participate, with the exception of four in Basel in 1967 and a much larger group in 1969 in Warsaw. It was necessary at that time to belong to a privileged group of so-called scientists with a travel permit to the non-socialist countries, which many could obtain only after many years of effort. The fact that Inna Nitz was able to participate in most of our annual meetings has to do with the unusual coincidence that she held a passport from the People's Republic of China.

Scientifically, the group was engaged in working out standardized recommendations for the most frequently performed X-ray examinations. These then became mandatory procedures. The first German monograph on ultrasound diagnosis was published in 1981, as was a monograph on skeletal dysplasias by E. Rupprecht and an atlas for bone age determination (hand) by Thiemann and Nitz. After German unification in 1990 this group dissolved. In the different regions of Germany, there are many regional working groups of paediatric radiologists who have regular meetings. Thus in the new states the former "GDR" group continues, together with Berlin, to hold two annual work sessions per year at which case presentations are discussed.

Centres for Paediatric Radiology in Germany

A short overview follows on the most important centres of paediatric radiology throughout Germany. There are, however, a good number of other departments/divisions of paediatric radiology, some in university hospitals and some in free-standing paediatric institutions.

Berlin

Whereas the first X-ray installation in a European children's hospital was set up in 1897 in Graz, Austria, the first one in Germany was installed in 1903 by Heubner at the famous Charité Hospital in Berlin. Until 1964 the the more experienced paediatricians were responsible for interpreting films and fluoroscopy results until Dieckhoff, then professor of paediatrics, appointed Inna Nitz, a fully trained radiologist, to be in charge of the X-ray department. Renate Kursave was put in charge of the X-ray installation for the paediatric surgical division in 1981.

As a result of the post-war situation, with the division of the city into four sectors and the old Humboldt University being situated in the Soviet sector, a new "Free University" was founded in the American sector. The Charlottenburg clinic became the centre of the medical school and the "Kaiserin Auguste Victoria Haus (KAVH)" with a long tradition in paediatric research a university clinic. Two paediatricians took a very active interest in radiology early on. H. Schäfer and L. Stolowski, both paediatricians, were very active and both have participated in the Paris and Stockholm meetings. They later moved on, the former had become Head of Paediatrics at the Rittberg Children's Hospital in Berlin, the latter as Head of Paediatric Radiology at the Children's Clinic in Berlin-Wedding. H. J. von Lengerke became Head of Radiology at KAVH in 1968 after a 3-month training period in Basel. He was joined by T. Klemm and succeeded by H.J. Kaufmann in 1979 after moving to Münster. Kaufmann obtained independent academic and administrative status for this department, which became a very busy training centre. Once a month meetings were organised for all those interested in paediatric radiology throughout Berlin, also its Eastern parts. He was very active as editor of books (e.g. on the pelvis, the series *Progress in Paediatric Radiology*, *Contrast Media in Paediatric Radiology* and *The Integration of Modern Imaging Methods in Paediatric Radiology*). He organised the 1981 meeting of the GPR in Berlin and since 1987 an annual meeting for the full-time German paediatric radiologists on professional and organisational topics. In the future this department will be combined with that of the Children's Clinic Berlin-Wedding, which is under the direction of T. Riebel, who was trained by M. A. Lassrich and received a professorship in Hamburg.

Bremen

In the newly constructed children's clinic in Bremen in 1928, a fluoroscopy room was accessible to all physicians; X-ray diagnosis, however, was performed by radiologists 300 m away in the "radiation house". All paediatric patients had to be transported there, some in laundry baskets (Fig. 7, 1958). When L. Schall (Fig. 11) became the head of the children's clinic, E. Willich (Fig. 8, 1965) was put in charge of the paediatric radiology department. By 1958 a modern department had been installed. Willich was in charge until he moved to Heidelberg in 1969 and was succeeded by Hildegard Müller-Brinkmann until 1990. In 1968 the departments in Bremen and Cologne

The History of Paediatric Radiology in Germany

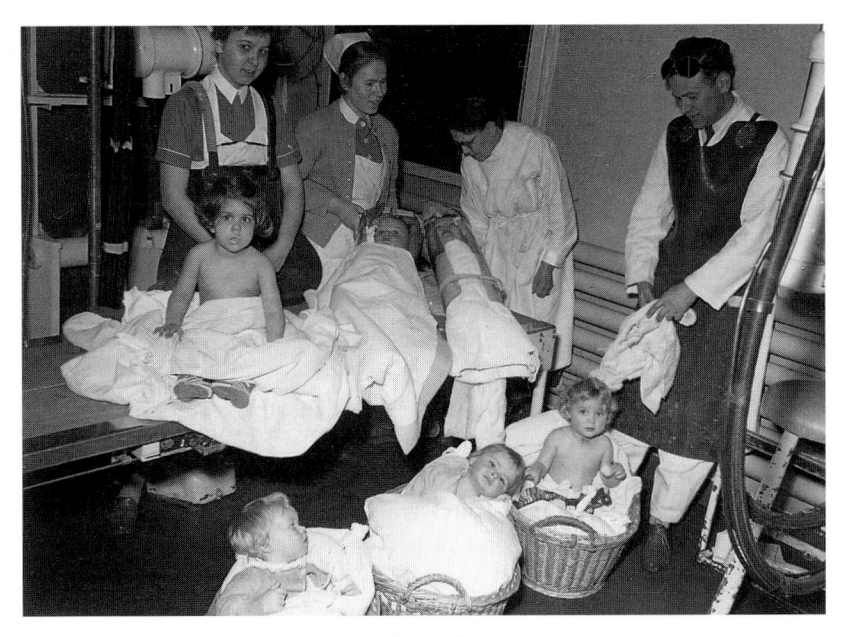

Figure 7
Transportation of small patients from the Children's Hospital Bremen to the "X-ray House" (1958). Wash baskets were used as transport containers for infants

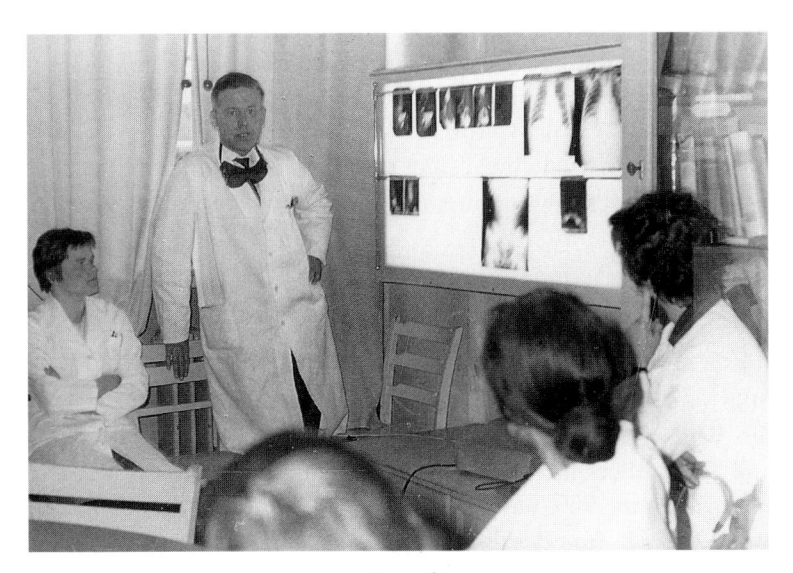

Figure 8
X-ray demonstration in the "X-ray House" in Bremen. E. Willich (1965)

(K.-D. Ebel and E. Willich), the book Röntgendiagnostik im Kindesalter (X-Ray Diagnosis in Childhood) was produced.

Cologne

The former Children's Clinic of the Medical Academy published contributions by F. Siegert, its director, on rickets (1903), mixoedema (1910) and chondrodystrophy (1912; 1914 also from E. Conradi) in the earliest days of X-rays. Together with Hünermann, the latter published in 1931 the first description of chondrodysplasia punctata; R. Grashey and F. Thoenes, well-known radiologists, were contributors to the first handbook on paediatric radiology by Engel and Schall (1933).

In 1962 a new children's hospital was opened by the city of Cologne. It had four chief physicians, one of whom was a paediatric radiologist: K.-D. Ebel (Fig. 11). This was to a large measure due to the efforts of H. Ewerbeck (died in 1987), later the president of the German Paediatric Society and an honorary member of the GPR. Ebel was a founding member of the ESPR and GPR. He was secretary of the GPR for 20 years and was very active professionally. In 1971 he organised the eighth meeting of the GPR', and in 1979 as president of ESPR organised its meeting in Cologne (Figs. 5 and 9). His department became quite reputable as a teaching centre, on an individual fellowship basis but even more so by having regularly offered training courses in paediatric radiology since 1985. In 1981 a subdivision of nuclear medicine was established after Ebel had spent some months with T. Treves in Boston. In 1982 a symposium was organised on "Paediatric Nuclear Medicine". Ebel retired in 1989 and was succeeded by his associate J. A. Bliesener.

Dresden

Since 1952, at the Children's Clinic of the Medical Academy in Dresden, children who could not be transported were examined with a portable machine. The others had to be moved 300 m to the X-ray department. Under Harnapp in 1959, one X-ray room was allocated to paediatrics. His successor Dietzsch appointed E. Rupprecht well known as a specialist of skeletal disorders, especially dysplasias, in 1968 as paediatric radiologist. In 1985 he received his professorship and is still in charge of this department.

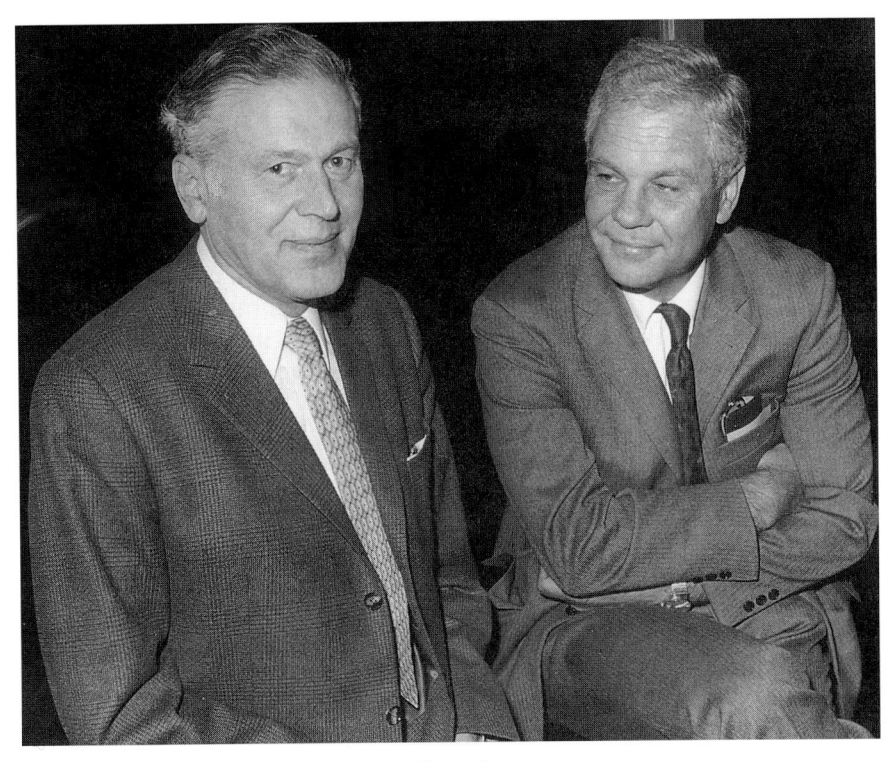

Figure 9
H. Fendel (†) and E. Willich. Paediatric Congress Cologne in 1976

Frankfurt am Main

By 1908 an X-ray room had been installed at the City Children's Clinic in Sachsenhausen. After the hospital became a university clinic in 1914, paediatricians performed their own radiological examinations. From 1948 on, O. Hövels, under De Rudder, was responsible for X-ray diagnosis. Modern installations were constructed in 1953. When Hövels became the Chief of Paediatrics in 1966, he appointed F. Ball to be in charge of paediatric radiology. From 1970 to his retirement in 1991, Ball headed the department. He organised the meeting of the GPR in 1972 and also the presentations when "imaging methods" were the main topic at the German Paediatric Congress in 1985.

Gießen

After publication of his monograph on the paediatric thorax, J. Duken gained renown in 1924. But it was not until 1972 that construction for a modern radiology department began in Gießen. One year later W. Schuster who was known from his work in Munich and Erlangen, was put in charge on the initiative of the paediatrician Dost and the cardiologist Rautenburg. Academically this department became quite important, producing a number of important publications – notably the two-volume German textbook on paediatric radiology in 1990. Three of his collaborators entered into academic careers: Prof. M. Reither now in Nuremberg, Prof. R. Schumacher now in Mainz and Dozent V. Klingmüller, still in Gießen.

Greifswald

In Greifswald under H. Brieger, an X-ray department has been in existence since 1950. It has been available to the most experienced paediatricians. Dr. Spiegelberg was in charge from 1960 to 1968, when Helga Wiersbitzky, a paediatric radiologist, took over. In 1973 this department became part of the university's radiology department so that access to nuclear medicine and later to ultrasound and CT became easier. H. Wiersbitzky was made professor in 1984 and organised the first international symposium on paediatric radiology in 1989 in the GDR.

Hamburg

A few years after World War II diagnostic radiological examinations were being performed in the destroyed buildings of the University Children's Clinic by M. A. Lassrich. From 1954 he was in charge of a new radiology department built under the direction of K. H. Schäfer. Lassrich, Schäfer and Prevôt published an atlas of paediatric radiology in 1955. In 1968 Lassrich organised in Hamburg the First ESPR Congress in Germany (Fig. 10). Hamburg was one of the most important centres for our speciality, often visited by physicians from Germany and abroad. This department was taken over in 1987 by E. Richter, who had been in charge at the Children's Hospital Altona.

The first department of paediatric radiology was established in the Children's Hospital Rothenburgsort, built in 1922. After the war this was one of the largest children's hospitals, comparable to Bremen and Leipzig with its more than 400 beds. From 1953 P. Siebert was full-time radiologist;

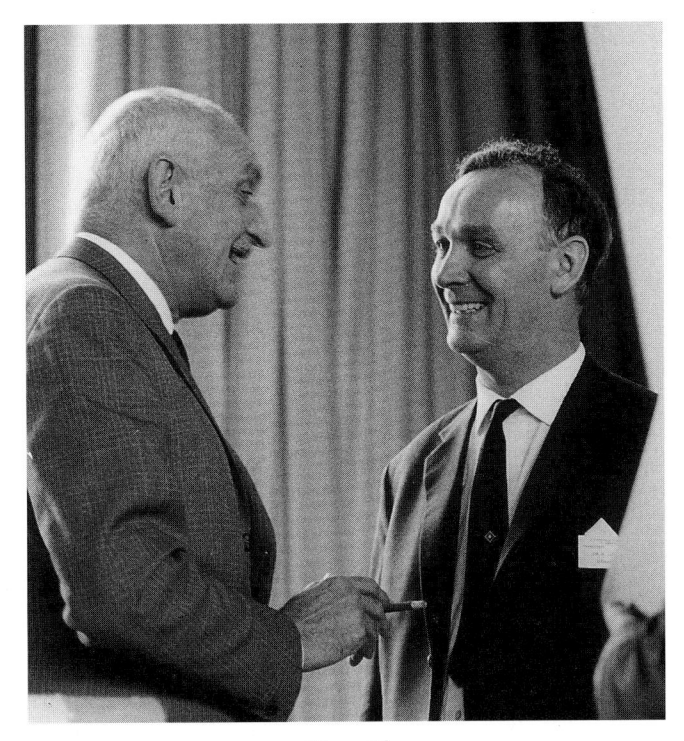

Figure 10
ESPR Congress Hamburg in 1968. J. Lefèbvre and M. A. Lassrich

in 1956 P. R. Koecher became the first chief physician of a paediatric radiologist department in Germany. From 1956 until this hospital was closed in 1982, W. Holthusen was the director of radiology. Subsequently, he was in charge of radiology at three different children's hospitals. He has written many scientific publications, and together with Lassrich organised the 1973 meeting of the GPR. Since 1987 he has been retired.

Heidelberg

The first X-ray equipment in Heidelberg was installed in 1921 at the "*Luisenheilanstalt*", which later became the University Children's Clinic, by W. Keller, later professor of paediatrics in Freiburg. From 1937 on J. Duken was in charge and as of 1948 until 1967 the paediatrician F. Schmid. When the clinic was reconstructed in 1965, a modern radiology department with three rooms was established. H. Bickel, who became professor of paediatrics in 1967, appointed E. Willich from Bremen (Figs. 6, 9 and 11) as director. Willich organised the annual GPR meeting 1969, received a professorship and was in charge until his retirement in 1984. Two of his associates who were awarded professorships, Gabriele Benz-Bohm and H. C. Oppermann, were later put in charge of the radiology department at the University Children's Clinics of Cologne and Kiel. Numerous publications are evidence of the activities of this department, which was taken over by J. Tröger in 1984. It has been enlarged and is now attached to the radiology department.

Leipzig

After Berlin, Leipzig was next to receive an X-ray department in 1903 which was staffed in the decades to follow by paediatricians and paediatric surgeons. When A. Peiper became professor of paediatrics (1948–1958), L. Weingärtner, who had participated in numerous ESPR congresses, was put in charge. He later became professor of paediatrics in Halle. The paediatric surgeon F. Meissner (1958–1988) took initiative in 1969 to have a radiologist, D. Hörmann, put in charge of the radiology department. Since 1976 Hörmann has also been responsible for the children's clinic. Between 1973 and 1990 he organised seven meetings of the paediatric radiology group of the former GDR in Leipzig and had responsibility for organising speakers and topics when paediatric radiology was the main theme of the 1987 Leipzig Congress of the radiological society of the former GDR (main speaker: H.J. Kaufmann).

Mainz

The University of Mainz was reactivated in 1946. Two years later the person to become professor of paediatrics, M. Köttgen, was one who had submitted a thesis on a topic in paediatric radiology. He installed an X-ray room so that children did not have to be transported to the central X-ray department anymore. In 1958 Sabine Wagner was the first paediatric radiologist to be employed, followed a year later by Irmgard Greinacher (see Fig. 5 in the chapter on Poland). Under her direction this department grew in size and importance but also in staff (three co-workers). The importance of ultrasonography was recognised early and introduced in 1974. A main area of interest was the skeleton when J. Spranger took over the paediatrics department. After I. Greinacher retired in 1988, R. Schumacher became its chief.

Munich

After 1950 radiology at the "Von Haunerschen Children's Hospital" was in the hands of general paediatricians and of the surgeon Prof. Fetzer. The institution had become the University Children's Hospital. In 1963 the head of the clinic, A. Wiskott, put W. Schuster in charge of radiology. When Schuster moved to Erlangen in 1966, C. Hager and Dr. Tamaela (Indonesia) continued his work until H. Fendel (Fig. 9) and K. Bethke from Tübingen moved to Munich (1976 and 1977). The former succeeded in making the radiology department an important centre, serving the paediatric and paediatric surgery departments. He introduced nuclear medicine and published widely. Internationally, he had considerable impact through the foundation of the "Lake Starnberg Group" and connections he had built up with the E.C., WHO and ESPR. The highlight of his career was the presidency of the ESPR and a perfectly organised ESPR meeting in Munich in 1990. Six months later he retired. But most unfortunately he died in 1991 of a malignant disorder. He was succeeded by K. Schneider. A second department of paediatric radiology was set up in 1971 at the Children's Clinic of the Technical University. This department is also responsible for paediatric surgery. D. Färber (Assistant professor), who was secretary of the GPR for 10 years, is head of this department; he also organised the annual meeting of the GPR in 1978.

Stuttgart

One of the last large German childrens' hospitals to receive its own radiology department was that in the Türlenstraße in Stuttgart. The head of this clinic, Grundler, appointed R. D. Schulz from Düsseldorf to become fulltime chief of radiology in 1971. However, in 1979 the clinic had to be closed and was integrated into the Olga Children's Hospital. Schulz was integrated into the radiology department there as head of special procedures and ultrasound diagnosis. He built up his new division to become the main place for training in paediatric ultrasound and with 11 000 examinations per year, it achieved great importance. Together with U. Willi, Zürich, he published an atlas on paediatric ultrasound.

As early as 1969, Helmut Hauke was put in charge of the radiology department at the Olga Children's Hospital. He was reponsible not only for internal paediatric medicine, but also for the surgical and ENT divisions, orthopaedics and traumatology. Since R. D. Schulz joined the department, it has grown into the largest department of paediatric radiology in Germany, with eight physicians, 12 technicians and seven other employees. Hauke is also in charge of radiological diagnosis in paediatric cardiology, and in 1990 the most modern equipment was installed here. He was in charge of the annual GPR congress in 1976, a function fulfilled by Schulz in 1983. As the teaching institution of the University of Tübingen, this department has achieved considerable repute.

Tübingen

In 1921, Lutz Schall, then a young fellow, was given the task by Professor W. Birk of setting up an "X-ray room". Schall describes his activities of the time as follows: "The explosion-like noise of the spark inductors which always occurred just at the moment when a child had been pacified, a strange smell of ozone and gas which emanated from the leaking interruptor, and the X-ray tube which was as temperamental as a spoiled woman and had to be set purely by instinct after each exposure were daily predicaments!".

Together with Birkner, Schall wrote a monograph in 1932 on the therapy of paediatric disorders using ultraviolet light and X-rays. In 1933, together with S. Engel, he edited the first handbook of paediatric radiology. In 1957, one of the first full-time positions as paediatric radiologist was created, and was given to Helmut Fendel (who later moved to Munich, Fig. 9). He made a name for himself in numerous important contributions (on carpometry) at congresses and in journals. From 1977 until his early death (1988), K. Nolte was in charge of the department.

Summary

Paediatric radiology in Germany has a very long tradition which goes back to the turn of the twentieth century. Initially, paediatricians carefully investigated the use of X-rays in paediatric diseases. There were many publications on the subject, only very few of which came from radiologists.

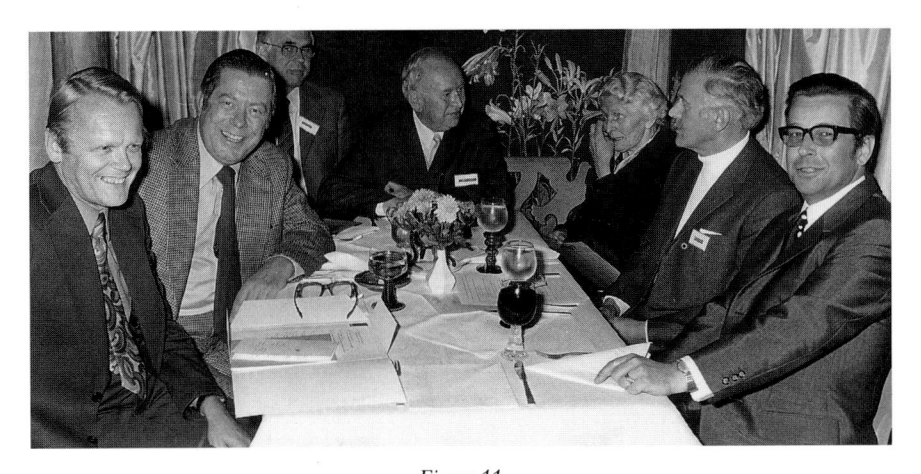

Figure 11
The last reunion around Lutz Schall: GPR Congress 1974 Würzburg (from the left): K.-D. Ebel, H. G. Wolf from Vienna (†), W. Menger, L. Schall (†), Mrs. Schall (†), E. Willich and D. Felsenreich

After World War II, notably M. A. Lassrich, H. Fendel, K. D. Ebel and E. Willich made lifelong careers in this field (Fig. 11). The were joined later by W. Schuster, F. Ball and H. Hauke. The development of paediatric radiology, now a subspeciality of radiology, in Germany was multicentric, and the division of Germany did not hinder its development. The integration of the former East German section of paediatric radiology into the GPR has now brought its membership to 290.

Paediatric Radiology in Great Britain and Ireland

E. Sweet

Early Paediatric X-Rays

In 1896, a 6-month-old boy was the subject of one of the earliest X-ray examinations in Britain. Dr. John McIntyre, an ear, nose and throat surgeon, demonstrated a coin lodged in his oesophagus, using a machine constructed in the Electro-Medical Department of the Glasgow Royal Infirmary. Within 15 years of Röntgen's discovery, most children's hospitals in Britain seem to have had X-ray machines, the responsibility of Medical Electricians or Radiologists, but the interpretation of the films produced was the prerogative of the paediatrician or surgeon looking after the patient. This failure to recognise the role of the radiologist in diagnosis continued for many years – cynics claim it still continues, citing the general lack of acknowledgement for diagnostic procedures throughout medical literature.

Radiology as a Specialty

Lack of recognition in the medical profession that the skill of ensuring adequate X-ray production should be combined with interpreting the resultant films led to the formation of what is now the Royal College of Radiologists, where ordinary membership is confined to medical practitioners. The College is responsible for devising training programmes, for accrediting training departments, for running the Fellowship examination (taken 3–4 years after starting full-time training in radiology), and for accreditation of Radiologists on completion of a recognised training programme. Other groups were formed earlier, but the Radiological Section of the Royal Society of Medicine was initially deemed to be too much under the influence of senior physicians and surgeons, and the British

Institute of Radiology admitted to membership physicists, radiographers and leaders of the X-ray manufacturing industry as well as radiologists, as it does today.

Paediatric Radiology as a Specialty

Recognition of specialty groups within both radiology and paediatrics is a relatively new phenomenon within Great Britain and Ireland and post-dates the establishment of the ESPR. Paediatric radiology owes its present status to the enthusiasm of individual members of the ESPR who were inspired by meeting their European colleagues, recognising the advantages of regular exchanges of ideas and of lasting friendships made across the world. When the National Health Service was established in 1948, most designated paediatric radiologists had much less than a full-time commitment to paediatric radiology, and Dr. Roy Astley was the first full-time paediatric radiologist appointed – to Birmingham Children's Hospital in 1948. Paediatric radiologists work in children's hospitals or in paediatric units within large hospital complexes serving children as well as adults, with shared apparatus but with examinations ideally, but not invariably under the control of paediatric radiologists. At present, the Hospital for Sick Children, Great Ormond Street, London, is the only self-contained children's hospital with all diagnostic services available on site. The Alder Hey Hospital in Liverpool will soon become the second, but all others are dependent on nearby hospitals dealing primarily with adults for at least one diagnostic service.

Paediatric Radiology Training

The adoption of multiple-choice examination techniques for the Fellowship examination helped the recognition of paediatric radiology as a sub-specialty. Paediatric radiology was the source of most of the examination questions, and trainees became enthusiastic about training – in opportunities! This led the Warden of the College to invite Dr. R. K. Levick to set up the Specialist Group of the Royal College of Radiologists in 1976 to advise on training. Following acceptance of the 1980 report from this group of senior paediatric radiologists, the College recommended a minimum of 3 months' practical training in paediatric radiology for all trainees in radiology and proposed that opportunities should be available for all those requesting post-fellowship training with a view to becoming paediatric radiologists. There is no statutory training requirement, and paediatric radiologists have to be accredited radiologists; experience in paediatrics is not essential, but desirable. In recent years, in spite of severe financial constraints, the opportunities to widen experience within Britain have been taken and more trainees have been able to arrange visits to centres of excellence in Europa, Australia, South Africa and the United States. The deplorable general ignorance of foreign languages has limited the use of the nearest centres of excellence.

Subspecialisation Within Paediatric Radiology

Subspecialisation in areas within paediatric radiology is becoming commoner. Paediatric neuroradiology was performed largely by neuroradiologists, dealing with adults as well as children, before the acquisition of computed tomography apparatus, which has led to much greater involvement of paediatric radiologists. Paediatric cardiology is becoming the responsibility of cardiologists in many centres with the increased use of echocardiography, but nuclear medicine is perhaps moving the other way, with more paediatric radiologists running nuclear medicine departments in Britain than in other European countries. Interventional radiology is spreading rapidly, with paediatric radiologists taking over from surgeons in procedures involving many systems.

Academic Posts

No academic posts are available in paediatric radiology in Great Britain or Ireland, although most paediatric radiologists are honorary clinical lecturers within their training centres. This is a reflection of the few opportunities for academic careers in radiology in our countries.

National Paediatric Radiology Groups

Individual paediatric radiologists have always participated actively in the work of the Royal College of Radiologists and the Faculty of Radiology of the Royal College of Surgeons of Ireland, many as committee Members.

Both institutions have convened scientific meetings with sessions devoted exclusively to paediatric radiology. This happened frequently in the 1980s, when interest in paediatric radiology among all radiologists seemed to peak. However, since 1979 paediatric radiologists have met as a group, at first annually, but more recently twice a year.

Radiology Group of the British Paediatric Association

Dr. R.K. Levick, Sheffield, was invited in 1979 to convene a group of radiologists who were members of the British Paediatric Association to present papers at a scientific session during annual general meetings. The group comprised paediatric radiologists from teaching hospitals but gradually enlarged to include any radiologist expressing an interest in paediatric radiology. This was an important extension, as at least 50% of radiology in children is still performed by other than paediatric radiologists in both Great Britain and Ireland. Dr. Levick was succeeded as Convener by Dr. S.E.W. Smith, Leeds, in 1985. The meetings increased in number to two each year – the first to coincide with the British Association of Paediatrics Meetings, now held in Warwick, and the second in winter, the location varying based on invitations from members of the group to their place of work. Between 60 and 80 members attended these popular meetings, where there was lively discussion and controversy in the best ESPR tradition.

British Paediatric Radiology and Imaging Group

In 1991 the Radiology Group of the British Paediatric Association and the Paediatric Specialty Group of the Royal College of Radiologists (which had concentrated on training) amalgamated under this title, with Dr. David Pilling of Liverpool elected as first chairman. All those interested in paediatric radiology in Great Britain and Ireland are eligible for membership. Both paediatric radiologists and those with a lesser commitment are represented on the committee. This group sees as its function the maintenance of a high profile for paediatric radiology by supporting members efforts to raise standards and increase knowledge. The meetings will continue to be held twice yearly.

Influence of ESPR on Paediatric Radiology in Britain and Ireland

The importance of ESPR to British paediatric radiologists cannot be exaggerated, as it was the first forum at which they met as a group, became friends, and realised how much could be achieved by exchanging ideas among themselves and with colleagues from the rest of Europe and farther afield.

British Radiologists in the ESPR

When Drs. Neuhauser and Lefèbvre met to plan the first meeting, Dr. P. Franklyn of Bradford was training in Boston. She was charged with finding interested British radiologists and contacted Dr. T. Lodge of Sheffield, who provided the list of those to be invited to the preliminary meeting in 1963. Those who attended became founding members of ESPR and, with a few notable additions, attended the first official ESPR session in Paris in 1964. There were eight from London, two from Liverpool and Manchester and one foundation member each from Aberdeen, Bradford, Edinburgh and Glasgow. Interests were wide; Dr. L.G. Blair of London had written extensively on the chest; Dr. John Sutcliffe of London, Dr. Norah Walker of Liverpool, and Dr. Patricia Franklyn of Bradford shared a common interest in the skeletal system; Dr. John Hodson of London and later Hamilton, Ontario, was the leading authority on pyelonephritis; Dr. John Dow was a cardiac radiologist; Dr. Roy Astley of Birmingham was a pioneer in cineangiocardiography in children and the author of a well-accepted textbook on the alimentary tract in infancy. As word spread, other paediatric radiologists made strenuous efforts to attend ESPR congresses and some made worthwhile contributions. These included Dr. Alan Chrispin of London and later Nottingham, who carried on the good work on the chest from the Hospital for Sick Children with outstanding work on cystic fibrosis. He became European Managing Editor of the new journal *Pediatric Radiology* and his last paper before retirement was presented in Paris in 1983, on real-time nuclear magnetic resonance after work done with other colleagues in Nottingham, including Dr. Philip Small, who read the paper and who has succeeded Dr. Chrispin as Managing Editor of *Pediatric Radiology*. Dr. R.K. Levick of Sheffield presented, in Warsaw in 1969, the first paper on abdominal ultrasound, and then early papers on this followed from Great Britain; these interested Professor Lefèbvre, who stimulated the French interest which has since proved such an outstanding feature of recent Congresses. Dr. Anne Hollman of Glasgow was, in Budapest in 1992, the first British recipient of the Jacques Lefèbvre Memorial Prize for her paper on colour doppler imaging of the paediatric scrotum, and the good publicity this is receiving will undoubtedly make ESPR better known to other radiologists throughout Britain.

Of those who attended in 1963 and 1964, Drs. Blair, Fawcitt, Hodson, Stewart, Sutcliffe and Walker are deceased. Drs. Astley, Davis, Dow, Franklyn, Hajdu, Macleod, Rawson and Warwick have retired. Another early member who is also deceased is Dr. Ian Gordon of Bristol, co-author of the first short British textbook on paediatric radiology which proved really popular with all trainees.

In recent years, Dr. Helen Carty of Liverpool and Dr. Isky Gordon of London have made regular contributions on nuclear medicine, and Dr. Paul Thomas of Belfast is one of the speakers whose pithy papers always draw a large audience, eager to be amused as well as instructed.

ESPR Congresses

Congresses in Great Britain and Ireland have been successful. The postgraduate courses have proved particularly helpful in spreading the word on paediatric radiology and the enthusiasm of the trainees attending certainly has helped the acceptance of paediatric radiology as a specialty by other radiologists. Dr. John Sutcliffe was president of the first London Congress in 1966. Dr. Roy Astley's congress in Birmingham in 1973 was one which really succeeded in keeping costs down to attract junior radiologists. Dr. E. M. Sweet presided at the Glasgow Congress in 1985, Dr. Noel Blake in Dublin in 1989. The Dublin Congress was not only an outstanding social success; it also showed how Ireland and Northern Ireland work together in radiology, with Dr. Blake's major support coming from Dr. V. Donoghue in Dublin and Dr. P. S. Thomas in Belfast. Dr. Thomas will be European co-president for the IPR'96 in Boston. In 1993 the Congress is to be held in London with Dr. Don Shaw as president. His contribution to paediatric radiology in Great Britain is outstanding; he has been on committees of the Royal College of Radiologists for many years, involved particularly with the Fellowship examination. He is also Editor of the *British Journal of Radiology*, the journal of the British Institute of Radiology. He is in great demand as an outstanding teacher.

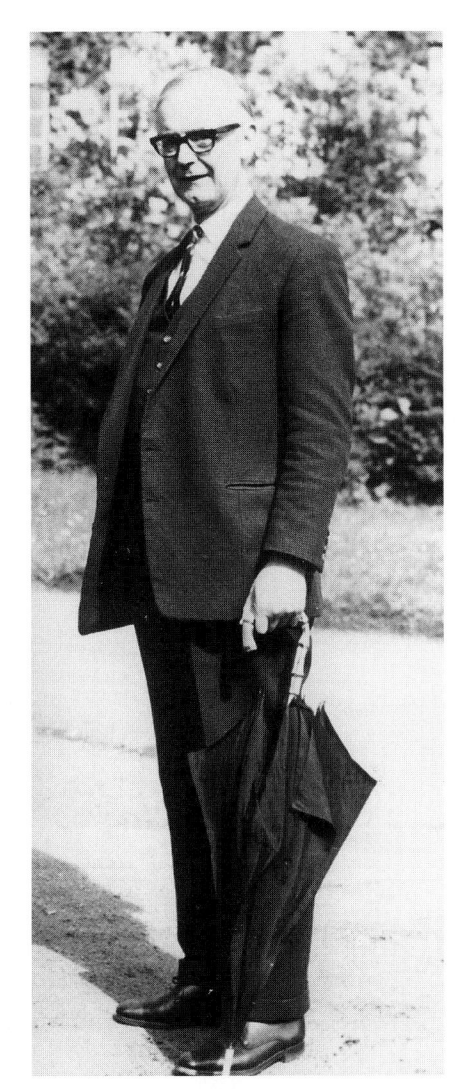

Figure 1
Dr. John Sutcliffe, President of the ESPR in 1966

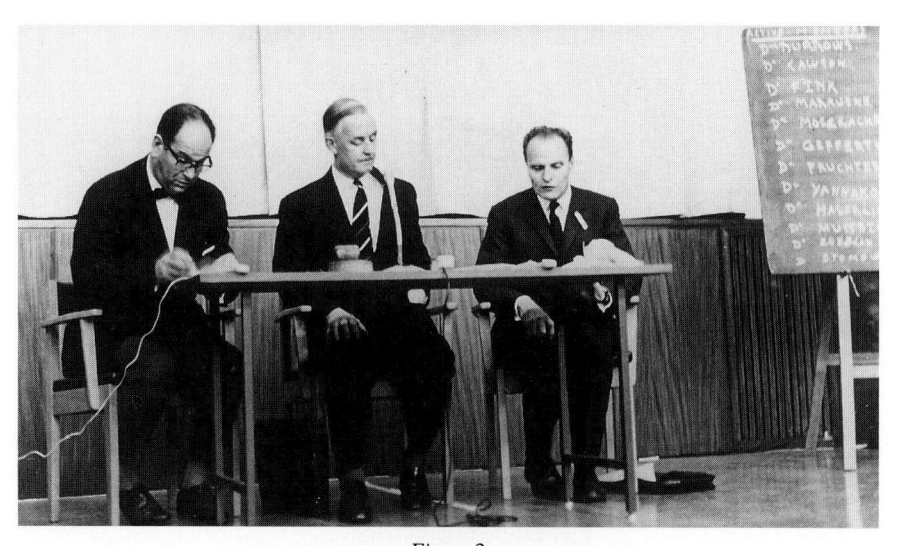

Figure 2
The chair at the business meeting of the ESPR in London in 1966. Note the names of new active members on the blackboard. From the left: J. Sauvegrain, J. Sutcliffe and H.J. Kaufmann

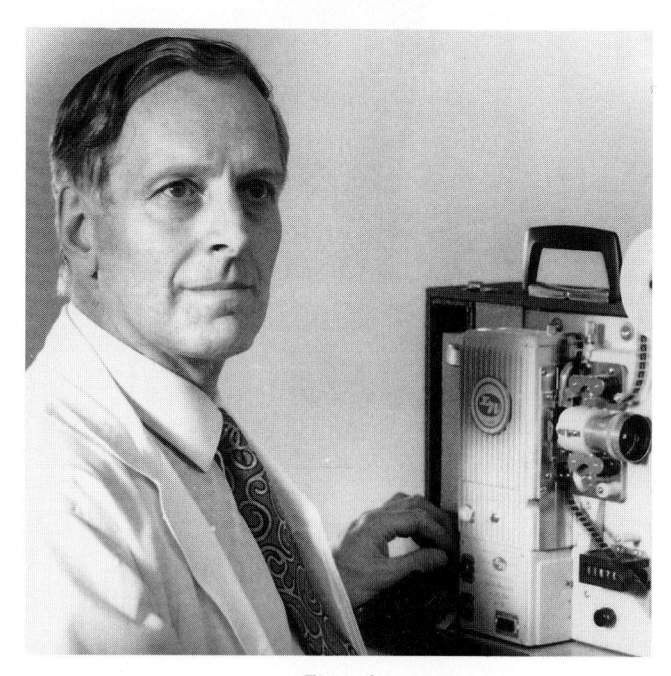

Figure 3
R. Astley, President of the ESPR and organiser of the Birmingham meeting in 1973 – in full action

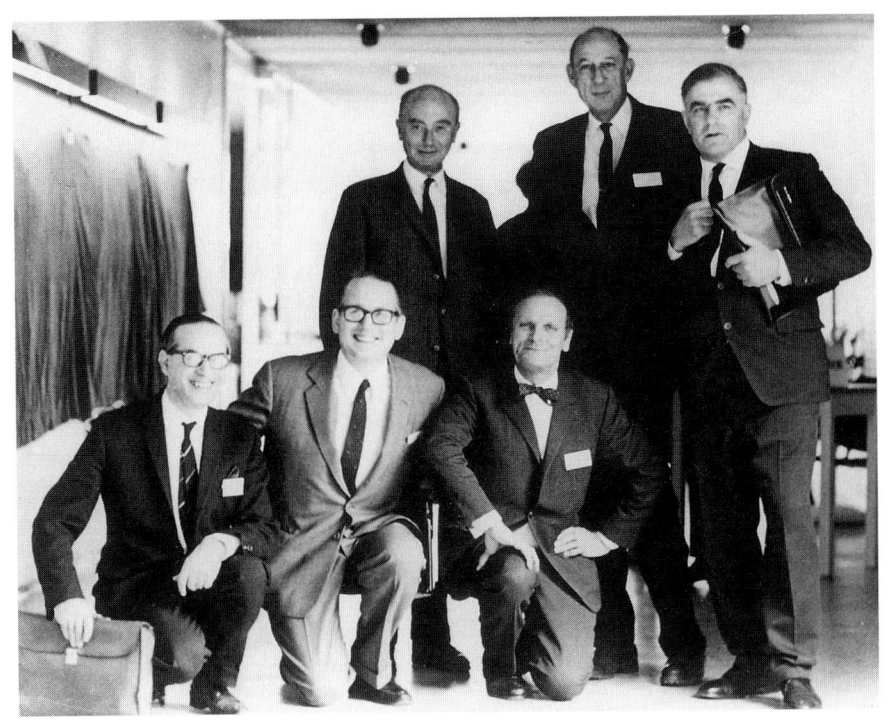

Figure 4
A happy group during intermission. Front row from the left: J. Sauvegrain, K. Knapp and P. Rawson. Standing: J. Hodson, E. B. D. Neuhauser and N. Hajdu

Conclusion

Although paediatric radiology is now recognised as a specialty by both paediatricians and radiologists, there are still fewer than 50 radiologists devoting most of their time to the specialty. They are scattered through the countries but now have a forum for continuing education and for planning concerted action to promote their needs, thanks to initiatives started by those who were founding members of the ESPR. Those of us working in Great Britain and Ireland owe a great debt to the European Society of Paediatric Radiology, which will continue to receive our strong support.

Acknowledgements. Most colleagues were supportive, but it was from Drs. Franklyn, Lamont, Levick, Smith, Stockdale and Thomas that I received the most help.

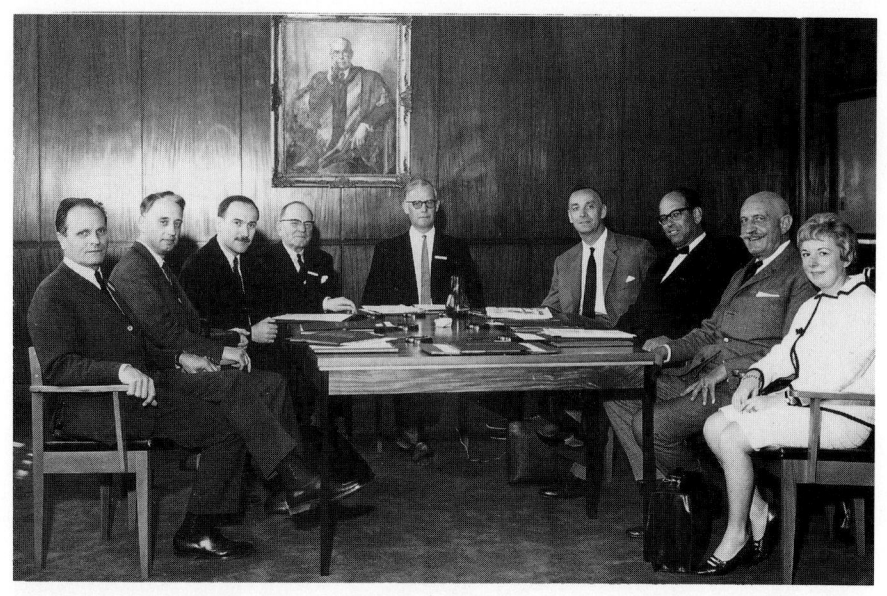

Figure 5
Meeting of the Executive Committee of the ESPR at the London Meeting 1966 from the left:
J. Sauvegrain, U. Rudhe, C. Fauré, L. G. Blair, J. Sutcliffe, A. Lassrich, H. J. Kaufmann,
J. Lefèbvre and Monique Fachard

References

Main books

1. Astley R (1956) Radiology of the alimentary tract in infancy. Arnold, London
2. Burrows EH (1986) Pioneers and early years, a history of British radiology. Colophon, Channel Islands
3. Gordon IRS, Ross FGM (1977) Diagnostic radiology in paediatrics. Butterworth, London

Topics of Selected Congress Papers

1963 Norah Walker, Liverpool, Peripheral dysostosis.
     John Hodson, London, Pyelonephritis.
1964 Roy Astley, Birmingham, Small intestinal pattern in some diseases.
1965 Roy Astley, Birmingham, Ventricular septal defects with infundibular stenosis.
1969 Keith Levick, Sheffield, Abdominal ultrasound.
1983 Philip Small and Alan Chrispin, Echoplanar imaging, real time nuclear magnetic resonance.
1992 Anne S. Hollman, Glasgow, Colour doppler imaging of the acute paediatric scrotum.

The History of Pediatric Radiology in Hungary

K. GEFFERTH, E. SCHLÄFFER and B. LOMBAY

The Beginnings [1]

In 1898 three articles concerning pediatric radiology were published in the journal *Medical Weekly*. One was written by Géza Faludy and illustrated by an X-ray picture taken by Károly Kiss, an assistant at the Technical University of Budapest. In all probability they obtained an X-ray machine from the Stephany Hospital where Faludy worked, because by 1900 Faludy and Deutsch were already reporting on regularly performed X-ray examinations.

Mihály Horváth, head physician of a general hospital, demonstrated hip dislocations with four photographs in 1901. Two years later Béla Alexander illustrated a lecture on the development of the spine with X-ray pictures. He published a monograph on this subject in 1906. By 1905 Jenő Kopits was performing follow-up X-ray examinations on patients with dislocation of the hip. Children with leukemia were being irradiated by Ármin Flesch in 1905, as were tuberculotic lymph nodes by János Bókay in 1906. A central X-ray unit was established at the Medical University of Budapest in 1907 under the direction of Béla Alexander, who wrote an excellent thesis on congenital lues in 1915.

In the Stephany Hospital the old X-ray machine, the origin and the quality of which remains unknown, was replaced by a new one in 1923. This was constructed by V. Szieghardt entirely from Hungarian materials, except for the high-tension wires, and was in use until it was replaced by a Siemens machine with a rotatory current regulator by J. Végh in 1955.

Prof. Bókay was aware that radiology could not merely be carried out as a secondary or subordinate activity and asked Prof. Kelen, head of the University Central Röntgen Institute, to send him an experienced radiologist as a consultant. This is how P. Mészöly began his career in 1925. By

---

[1] This section was written by K. Gefferth †.

the following year two papers had been published by him in the newly launched Hungarian radiologic journal (1926). In the same issue there were other papers concerning pediatric radiology: one by O. Göttche (1926) from the Pediatric Department of the University of Pécs, and another by J. Gajzágó (1926) from the University Gynecology Hospital in Budapest. The latter author referred to a newborn baby with chondrodystrophy, and, judging by the photo, by the radiograph and by the clinical course, this may be seen as the first case of thanatophoric dysplasia in the literature. A. Horváth (1926) dealing with anomalies of the urinary tract reports on the case of an 18-month-old infant with renal anomaly.

At this time the X-ray department of the Stephany Hospital moved to the second floor into a 32 m^2 room in which one corner was partitioned off as the darkroom. The remaining area was divided into two parts by a portable wall covered with lead. One of them was used for fluoroscopy and the other one for radiography and therapy (Fig. 1 a, b). The physician in charge did all the work, including registration of patients, preparing handwritten reports, developing films, etc. Patients were undressed and prepared for examination in the same room. The main constituent of the work was fluoroscopy and a 10-min period of adjusting to the darkness was required, as total darkness was necessary in the room. Infants were placed in a Wimberger chair; their hands and feet were held by an accompanying person. The fluoroscopy screen hanging on two strings had to be fixed by hand. As an electrical cable was hanging free in the room, great care was required to avoid electrocution. A long lead apron and lead gloves were worn during fluoroscopy and a shorter apron was worn by the assistant. Radiographs were usually made on films or on papers, which were less expensive.

Károly Gefferth joined the clinic in 1930, working there as a subordinate until Pál Meśzöly left. Gefferth became a radiologist in 1933, qualified as a lecturer in 1948 and became a Candidate of the Academy in 1956. He remained at the clinic until his retirement in 1971 (Fig. 2).

In the 1930s the hospital acquired a modern X-ray machine which was placed in an 8.4 m^2 room under the supervision of Péter Sonnauer. He chose to perform not only diagnostic work, but rather X-rayed patients according to their needs. György Köteles joined the laboratory in 1956 and stayed until 1958 when, at the invitation of Pál Kemény, he transferred to the Madarasz Street Hospital. He was succeeded by Edit Rokay on 1 January 1959.

In 1948 the X-ray laboratory moved into its own building where the areas for photography, radiography and therapy were separated. Radiation protection was taken care of by the exacting work of Gyula Koczkás, the

The History of Pediatric Radiology in Hungary

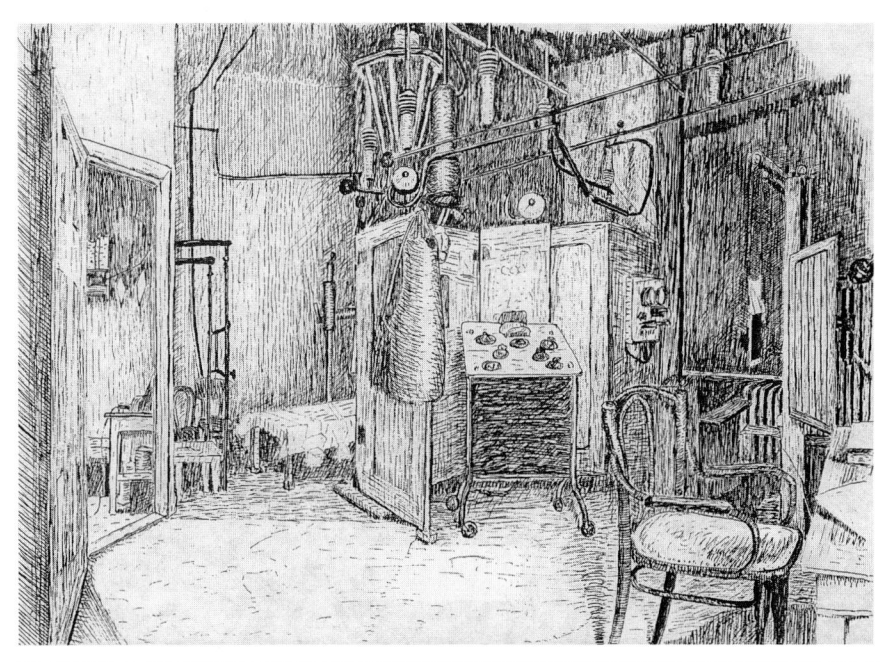

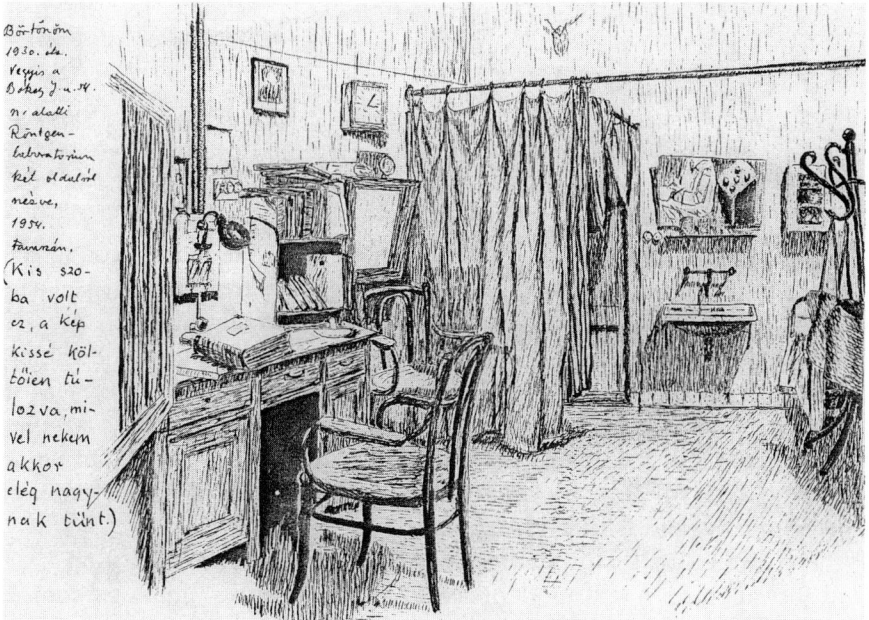

Figure 1
The X-ray department of the Stephany hospital

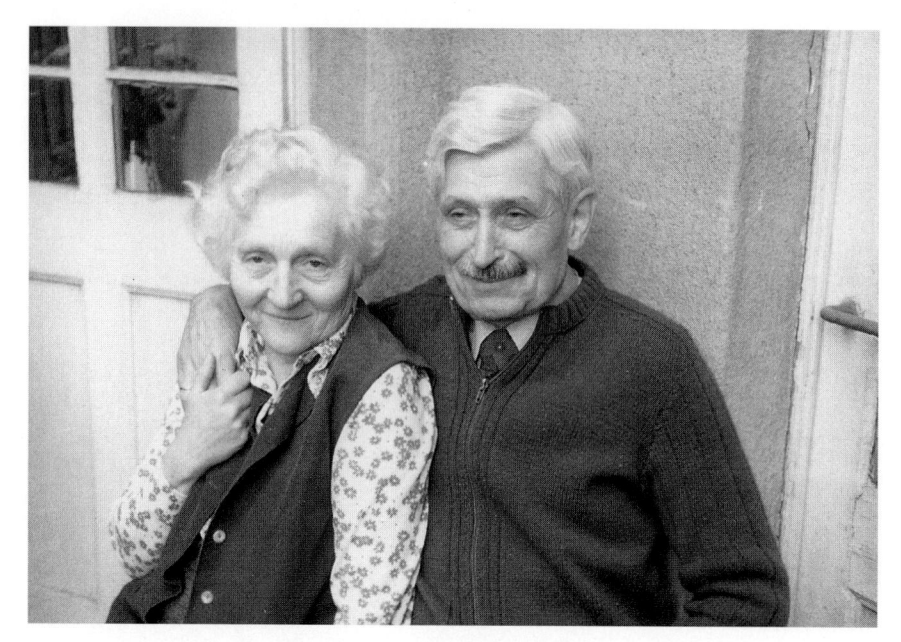

Figure 2
Károly Gefferth (1901–1992) and Mrs. Gefferth

electrical engineer. The Swiss Red Cross presented a four-valve Müller apparatus to the hospital which was in use from 1957 onwards.

Görgényi-Göttche from Pécs began his pioneering radiological work at the Second Children's Clinic in Budapest in 1953. He did almost all the radiology work alone although he benefited greatly from the assistance of Zsebök in 1954 and Kassay in 1958. Hungarian radiology was greatly encouraged by René Fonó who also performed much groundbreaking work with Imre Littmann in 1957. He also introduced a sheet changer for the provision of his heart patients. In 1953, Görgényi-Götche, as director of the State Children's Sanatorium in Szabadsághegy, expanded his work in the field of radiology by organizing 1½-day symposia. Ákos Görgényi headed the Second Children's Clinic.

The Szent László Hospital received their first X-ray apparatus in 1929 and the laboratory was modernized in 1940. Pediatric radiology took a significant step forward through the work of Vince Augusztin on measles and the lung in 1959; he had been head of the laboratory since 1948. In the same period László Binder (1954–1955) was also particularly active and his work on primary staphylococcus pneumonia and desinvaginations was of particular significance. Erzsébet Schläffer started her career working side-by-side with these people and stayed at Szent László until 1967 when she was appointed head of the X-ray section at the Apáthy István Children's Hospital.

In 1954 under the leadership of Károly Wattner the Pediatric Clinic in Szeged achieved outstanding results on plasma cell pneumonia; László Páldy made a name for himself at this time by systematizing X-ray alterations.

The Pediatric Clinic in Pécs received Phillips equipment in 1944. Since 1933 Oszkár Göttche had worked there; he contributed two chapters to the paediatric radiology handbook by Engel and Schall. In 1948, Ferenc Varga wrote about Thiemann-Fleischner's disease. The experienced specialist János Weisenbach succeeded Oszkár Lombos and Ignác Kopcsányi as head of the laboratory.

By 1937 the Debrecen Pediatric Clinic already had an X-ray machine, paid for by the physicians themselves. The pediatricians took their own X-rays. From the beginning of the 1950s there was a separate X-ray laboratory staffed by a head assistant and radiology specialists.

In 1929 a Children's Hospital was opened in Budapest's Madarasz Street with Ármin Flesch as the senior consultant – a man famous for his work with X-rays of the infant's stomach (1911). When he left in 1958 he was succeeded by Pál Kemény, on whose initiative György Köteles joined the staff. Up until then the laboratory had functioned within quite narrow bounds, but Köteles supervised the subsequent development and modernization and his name is closely connected with a number of published articles and books.

We cannot possibly conclude our story without recalling Zsabök's (1960) achievement X-ray anatomy of the lung. Russmann's procedures developed for diagnosing mastoiditis in babies should also be remembered. In a broader, historic view of Hungarian and also international pediatric radiology Károly Gefferth (1944), János Biró (1953), and Béla Rossman (1956) were the key figures.

Modern Pediatric Radiology [2]

In the 1960s there was a worldwide revolution in the technical development of X-ray equipment. More and more new and modern machines

---

[2] This section was written by E. Schläffer and B. Lombay.

were adapted for pediatric practice, too, mainly in the developed countries. Unfortunately Hungary was not able to follow this trend and for several years stayed at the "old" technical level in both general and pediatric radiology. Despite the disadvantageous circumstances, there was progress in the scientific field thanks to Profs. Zoltán Zsebök and Mihály Erdélyi, directors of the Radiologic Clinic and Postgraduate Medical School, Department of Radiology in Budapest. Meetings and consultations for pediatric radiologists were held regularly in the Postgradute Medical School in Budapest and in other clinics in the country.

A milestone in the history of Hungarian pediatric radiology was reached in 1977. By accepting the suggestion of Dr. Erzsébet Schläffer the Pediatric Radiology Section was established as a body of the Hungarian Radiological Society. Dr. Schläffer was the first president of the Section and later was reelected twice for two 4-year terms. During this period there were about 60 members in the Section, most of whom had specialized in both pediatrics and radiology with a special interest in new methods and results of radiology. Regular meetings and postgraduate courses were organized in special fields of pediatric radiology and more and more papers and books were published on such topics. Because there were only a few special books in Hungary at that time, these became indispensable for daily practice. The need for pediatric radiology by general radiologists dealing with pediatric patients and the influence of the development of pediatric radiology in the developed countries forced the establishment of pediatric radiology teaching centers in Hungary. At the beginning, these existed in technically very modest circumstances but the radiologists in charge were very skilled and enthusiastic. Some centers and their chiefs were: First Pediatric Clinic with Sándor Szy, Second Pediatric Clinic with Akos Görgényi in Budapest; Madarász Children's Hospital with György Köteles, Pál Heim Children's Hospital with Judit Madarász, and Apáthy Children's Hospital with Erzsébet Schläffer in Budapest; furthermore, the Pediatric Clinic with László Páldy and József Beviz in Szeged; Pediatric Clinic with János Weisenbach and Children's Hospital with Ignác Kopcsányi in Pécs; Pediatric Clinic with Aniko Makai in Debrecen; and Child Health Center with Magdolna Ormóshegyi and Matild Németh in Miskolc.

The newest institution, with more than 500 pediatric beds and all the subspecialities of pediatrics, is the Clinic of the Postgraduate Medical University in Miskolc which was established in 1976; it has all the facilities required for modern diagnosis and treatment. This institute offers regular postgraduate courses every year.

Because of the unfavorable political circumstances, the activities of pediatric radiologists in that era were hindered by rigorous regulations concerning travel abroad. Permission for someone to participate in a congress organized in a Western country was considered to be an extra favor from the government. Fortunately there were very reliable colleagues in the Western countries who during these difficult times helped their Hungarian counterparts, offering not only possibilities but also gracious donations as well. The Section is very grateful to the Gesellschaft für Paediatrische Radiologie (GPR) and its former president Professor Eberhard Willich for their generous assistance and also to Dr. Elizabeth Sweet in Glasgow who welcomed us to the European Society of Pediatric Radiology. Both are honorary members of the Hungarian Radiologists' Society. The Section has very good contacts with the European Society; one honorary member and five active members are working for the ESPR. Since the early 1980s, besides several domestic meetings, the Section has had the opportunity to organize international meetings every 2 years, with participants from both East and West. The X-ray Department of the Pediatric Clinic in Pécs and the Child Health Center in Miskolc undertook the organization. These meetings became very popular and flourished, forming a bridge between East and West.

In addition in 1988 an annually published English-language international journal *Year Book of Pediatric Radiology* was founded. Its aim is to provide an opportunity to publish articles by colleagues not only from Hungary but from anywhere in the world. It has proved to be a great success.

We hope that the changes going on at the moment will go a long way to improve our capabilities here at home and the world in general.

Bibliography

Alexander B (1906) Entwicklung der knöchernen Wirbelsäule. Gräfe and Sillem, Hamburg
Alexander B (1915) Die ossealen Veränderungen bei kongenitaler Syphilis. J. Barth, Leipzig
Augusztin V, Binder L (1955a) Segmentale Röntgenschatten bei Pertussis. Monatsschr Kinderheilkd 103:409–411
Augusztin V, Binder L (1955b) Segmentale Röntgenschatten bei Pertussis. Fortschr Geb Röntgenstr Nuklearmed 83:353–365
Binder L (1955) Die Röntgensymptome der primären Staphylokokkenpneumonien im Säuglingsalter. Fortschr Geb Rontgenstr Nuklearmed 82:584–590
Fényes I, Zoltán L (1959) Calvé's disease: does it exist? The question of its aetiology. Br J Radiol 32:394–403
Fonó R, Littmann I (1957) Die kongenitalen Fehler des Herzens und der großen Gefäße. Diagnostik und operative Behandlung. Barth, Leipzig
Gefferth K (1942) Beiträge zur Röntgentherapie der Hautkrankheiten im Säuglings- und Kleinkindesalter. Kinderarztl Prax 13:147–149

Gefferth K (1948) Über Empfindlichkeit der kindlichen Haut gegenüber Röntgenstrahlen. Kinderarztl Prax 16:42–46

Göttche O (1931) Säuglingssattel für Röntgenuntersuchung der Säuglinge. Rontg Prax 3:137–140

Göttche O (1933) Chronisch nicht spezifische Lungenerkrankungen. In: Engel – Schall (ed) Handbuch der Röntgendiagnostik und Therapie im Kindesalter. Thieme, Leipzig

Göttche O (1933) Röntgenuntersuchung der kindlichen Tuberkulose. In: Engel – Schall (ed) Handbuch der Röntgendiagnostik und Therapie im Kindesalter. Thieme, Leipzig

Görgényi-Göttche O, Zsebök Z (1954) Die Bedeutung der frontalen Schichtbilder in der Röntgendiagnostik der Lungentuberkulose vom Erwachsenen-Typ im Pubertätsalter. Mod Prob Pädiatr 1:518–526

Görgényi-Göttche O, Kassay D (1958) Atelektasen im Kindesalter. Erg Ges Tuberkulose Lungenf 14:391–479

Páldy L (1965) Neues Hilfsgerät zur radiologischen Diagnose der Säuglinge und Kleinkinder. Radiol Diagn (Berlin) 6:349

Rossmann B (1957) Einfache Aufnahmetechnik des Säuglingsohres. Fortschr Geb Rontgenstr Nuklearmed 86:741–748

Waltner K, Diósszilágyi G, Páldy L, Török J, Koltay M (1954) Die interstitielle Pneumonie der Frühgeborenen. Klinischer Teil. Acta Med Hung 5:371–402

The History of Pediatric Radiology in Hungary

The Pioneers of Pediatric Medicine *

Károly Gefferth

Károly Gefferth was born in Újkécske (about 120 km southeast of Budapest on the River Tisza) on 28 January 1901. His father was a general practitioner, and he began his own course of study in medicine in the Faculty of Medicine at Pázmány Péter University in Budapest at the age of 17 years, gaining his doctorate in 1924. After first working as a doctor in Budapest, Gefferth worked for a long time in Germany (in Tübingen and Heidelberg, and in Cologne with Werner Teschendorf), concentrating on paediatrics and, especially, roentgenology. From October 1930 to November 1971, Gefferth then worked in the 1st Department of Paediatrics at the University Hospital in Budapest, with a break during World War II when he had to take charge of a hospital in Szekesfehervar (Weissenberg). In 1933 he qualified formally as a roentgenologist, and in 1948 as a lecturer with his thesis: *Pädiatrische Aspekte der Röntgenologie* (paediatric aspects of roentgenology).

Gefferth is one of the pioneers of paediatric roentgenology. Over the course of half a century, in a good 125 publications in both radiology and paediatrics journals, in chapters contributed to multi-author works and in monographs, he has dealt with virtually the whole range of roentgenology in that timespan, supplementing and extending it. His publications – most of them one-man productions but some team efforts, mostly under his direction – have appeared, predominantly in radiology and paediatrics journals published in his homeland, but many appeared in *Fortschritte auf dem Gebiete der Röntgenstrahlen* and *Strahlentherapie* and also in the big German paediatrics journals. (Gefferth published in Hungarian, German, English and French.) Whatever the topic – studies relating to colonic relief in infants or other imaging procedures applied to the abdominal organs, roentgenological questions connected with heart defects and pulmonary or pleural illnesses, congenital or acquired changes in the skeletal system, irradiation risks and protection in infants and children or any other subjects relating to both paediatrics and roentgenology – Gefferth's name crops up in the relevant literature. He elaborated the procedure for roentgenological imaging of the mastoid in infants and described the roentgenological phenotypes of interstitial plasma cell pneumonia in prematures. He was concerned with the growing skull. He compiled ossification age tables (1968), a procedure for the determination of biological bone age (1970) and metric evaluation of the short tubular bones of the hand from birth up to the end of puberty. In 1968, his paper on metatropic dysplasia, a clinical picture that he later took up again in Volume 4 of *Progress in Pediatric Radiology*, appeared in *Zeitschrift für Kinderheilkunde*, the forerunner of *European Journal of Pediatrics*. In *Handbuch der Kinderheilkunde*, edited by H. Opitz et al., Gefferth described the clinical and radiological aspects of organ-localized and generalized moniliasis (Springer 1963); in *Perinatal Medicine*, edited by E. Kerpel-Fornius et al., he presented the radiology of the respiratory tract, of the abdominal organs and of diseases of the bones (Budapest 1978). As late as 1984 he published an original article on bone alterations during long-term remissions in leukaemic children.

Károly Gefferth is approaching his eighty-eighth birthday. Although he has already been retired for a long time, he continues to frequent his room in the paediatrics department of the university hospital; his lively interest in science is unabated; he still writes a clear hand; and he takes an enthusiastic interest in the specialist training of the more junior members of the hospital staff in roentgenology, devoting his considerable pedagogic talents to this end.

---

* Already published in *European Journal of Pediatrics 1988*, Vol. 148, pp 1–2.

All who are personally acquainted with Károly Gefferth value him highly as an exceptionally refined and distinguished character. They know he loves literature and the visual arts – especially painting – and is a connoisseur of both. He is also a great patriot. At the same time, however, he is a true European, indeed a cosmopolitan. In 1973 he was elected to honorary membership of the European Society of Pediatric Radiology, and he is also an honorary member of the Society for Pediatric Radiologists from German-speaking Countries, whose 1981 meeting in Berlin he attended at the age of 80.

International paediatrics owes Károly Gefferth both respect and gratitude.

H.-R. WIEDEMANN, Kiel

Paediatric Radiology in Italy: Its Status Before and After the Foundation of the European Society of Paediatric Radiology

G. BELUFFI

To write about paediatric radiology in Italy is not an easy task. In fact, I would say that in some respects it is very difficult, since the topic deals with what could be called a type of archeology, both on radiological and paediatric levels.

As in archeology, in order to investigate the history of paediatric radiology in Italy, one has to deal with ideas and information deriving from the memories of a few helpful colleagues. This information is at times very precise and correct, yet at other times quite vague. In addition, one often has to make desperate efforts in order to find the missing link, especially in such instances where memory and good will fail, or when nobody is available to help or give suggestions.

In Italy, most of the true paediatric hospitals were founded either as orphanages (the most famous being the *Spedale degli Innocenti* in Florence, designed by F. Brunelleschi in 1426 and completed in 1445 during the Renaissance), or as places for the very poor, who were attended to usually by nuns, a few nurses and perhaps an obliging doctor. The majority of these institutions were established as charities by wealthy people, generous citizens, noble families and the Church. They in turn provided funding to a variable degree. Even though these institutions were commendable for their efforts, they unfortunately suffered from the ups and downs naturally linked to such a financial background.

As examples, reference is made to the *Istituto per l'Infanzia e Pie Fondazioni Burlo Garofolo e Dott. Alessandro ed Aglaia de Manussi* in Trieste, founded in 1856; the *Ospedale Pediatrico* A. Meyer in Florence, founded in 1884; the *Ospedale dei Bambini* in Milan, founded in 1898 (this hospital is now called *Ospedale dei Bambini V. Buzzi* and also treats adult patients); the *Ospedale Bambino Gesu'* in Rome; the *Ospedale Regina Margherita* in Turin, and other *Ospedale dei Bambini* in Alessandria, Ancona, Brescia and Trento.

Completely different was the situation concerning paediatric departments within a general hospital, or paediatric clinics within a university hospital. All of these were organized as integrated wards in the hospital system, each with their own staff and each partaking of all the diagnostic opportunities offered within the hospital walls.

The *Istituto G. Gaslini* in Genoa, founded in 1937, can be considered to be half-way between all of the above, having been founded as a charity whilst maintaining very close connections with the University of Genoa's Departments of Paediatrics, which were and still are located within the hospital.

What, you may ask, has this long preamble to do with paediatric radiology? It has little, and yet so much to do with it: little, because we have not spoken about paediatric radiology yet; so much, because in some way, out of this peculiar system, paediatric radiology in Italy has developed.

At one moment or another it was indeed realized that not only a good clinician, proper medications or surgery were enough in the diagnostic evaluation and treatment of patients admitted to these hospitals. In some way or other diagnostic rooms for radiological purposes (called *Gabinetti Radiologici*) started to see the light (or rather the darkness!). The first was located in Bologna in the early 1920s (1922) at the *Ospedale Gozzadini's*, University Paediatric Clinics. This was under the direction of Dr. P. Sighinolfi, who later became chief radiologist at the *Ospedale Civile* in Ravenna.

In these early days, between the 1920s and early 1930s, these *Gabinetti Radiologici* were very often beyond the control of a radiologist. Instead, those in charge of them, who also personally took the films, were pediatricians or surgeons, if not outside volunteers.

When it was recognized by hospital administrations that a radiologist should be in charge of a *Gabinetto Radiologico*, the person nominated was either a general radiologist, who usually worked part-time, or a *consulente* (the consulting radiologist), who spent a few hours a day, or only a few a week there.

This change happened in Trieste in 1939, when A. D.'Agnolo was appointed Assistant Specialist in Radiology. In Milan it occurred in the late 1920s with Maria Pellini, first as *consulente*, then as chief of the Department of Radiology (*Ospedale Buzzi*). In Turin, G. M. Reviglio became *consulente* at the Regina Margherita Hospital in 1935 and later on was the first to be appointed Chief Radiologist, holding that position until 1968. In Genoa, the Section of Diagnostic Radiology started its work in 1937, at the same time at which the Gaslini Institute was officially opened. It was initially under the supervision of Prof. A. Vallebona, who held this position for many years, then from 1947 under Dr. G. Balestra who was the first to be officially chief of the department. He in turn was succeeded by A. De Maestri (1951–1959), followed by N. Maccarini (1962–1968) and then by A. Pelizza (1968 till the present day).

In Florence, E. Cumbo was the first *consulente* of the *Gabinetto Radiologico*, since 1946 associated with the University's Institute of Radiology. Thus, the radiologists who spent their time in the Section of Paediatric Radiology were always under the supervision and advice of the Director of the University's Institute of Radiology, who at that time was Prof. L. Turano. G. De Giuli was put in charge of the section in 1946 and held this position until 1953. He was succeeded by C. Bompiani until 1956, and then by G. F. Vichi, who became the first to be appointed as chief when the section was recognized as a fully independent structure in 1968.

In Rome, the *Ospedale del Bambino Gesu'*, previously an orphanage, officially opened in 1936. Its first *consulente* was L. Traversa, followed by M. Cesarini in 1958 and by P. Gugliantini from 1975 to 1991.

In Bologna P. Sighinolfi was the first *consulente*, followed by Giorgina Giacomini until 1951; by G. Golfieri during the 1960s; by C. Montanelli until 1983; and by A. Lucchi from 1983 to 1987.

In Naples the *Ospedali Riuniti per Bambini* was formed in the late 1930s by the merging of two hospitals (Pausilipon and Santobono) plus the heliotherapeutic centre "Attilio Curcio". Chief radiologist there from 1954 to 1973 was F. Soricelli. Due to the splitting of these hospitals in 1978, he was succeeded by C. Sandomenico at the Pausilipon (1975 onwards) and F. Cesaruolo at the Santobono.

Who were these *consulente*? They were general radiologists who, from one day to the next, found themselves entangled in a completely different sort of world. They were often "invited" to take up a position, if not simply sent to occupy a new post, by the professor of radiology. It was impossible to answer "no" to these requests, which were more often than not expectations, for endless reasons.

Some gave up very soon, but most stayed and became, without being aware of what was really happening, the true fathers of paediatric radiology in this country. A short list includes: Maria Pellini in Milan, G. M. Reviglio in Turin; A. D'Agnolo and A. Della Santa in Trieste, L. Traversa and M. Cesarini in Rome, G. Balestra and A. De Maestri in Genoa, E. Cumbo and G. De. Giuli in Florence. Under their guidance, training of other young radiologists began. These young radiologists (A. Pelizza in Genoa, P. Gugliantini in Rome, E. Schiavetti in Milan, G. F. Vichi in Florence, G. S. Marchese in Turin, C. Montanelli in Bologna, C. Sandomenico and F. Cesaruolo in Naples) worked in close contact with the pioneers. They became the link between the founders of paediatric radiology and the new era which was starting to see "the light" beyond the borders of the country.

Those were the days in which few papers were published (Pellini 1934, 1940; Bulgarelli e De Maestri 1952; De Giuli 1954; Bompiani 1957). Those were also the days in which no textbooks of general paediatric radiology were at hand, apart from monographs, such as the one on skull roentgenology (Lischi and Menichini 1959). At that time the first Italian translation of Caffey's book (1961) was a landmark.

The above can be considered to be the centres where a prototype for a "School of Paediatric Radiology" was established during the late 1950s and early 1960s. Yet, during the 1960s, there were still hospitals and paediatric clinics in which self-made paediatric radiologists emerged: G. Iannaccone in Rome (Paediatric Clinic of the University); F. Bellini in Milan (*Ospedale Istituti Clinici di Perfezionamento*); M. Pini in Trieste; and G. De Filippi, first in Trieste and later on in Alessandria, as the first chief radiologist in the local *Ospedale dei Bambini* (1973 onwards).

Prof. G. Currarino must be remembered here. After earning his degree in medicine at the University of Genoa in 1945, followed by 2 years of training in paediatrics under Prof. G. De Toni, he moved to the U.S.A. where his interest in paediatric radiology developed. He first trained under Prof. F.N. Silverman at the Children's Hospital in Cincinnati and then under Prof. E.D.B. Neuhauser in Boston. He was on the staff as a paediatric radiologist at the Children's Hospital in Cincinnati (1955–1960) and the New York Hospital (Cornell University, 1960–1965), and then became chief radiologist at the Children's Hospital, Dallas (University of Texas, in 1965).

In the 1960s the man who most certainly understood the importance of paediatric radiology in all its facets, but especially with regard to how it distinctly differs from adult radiology, was G.S. Marchese from Turin (Fig. 1). He was the first radiologist who tried to unite his colleagues, who had been working quite independently in their own hospitals, in order to form what was called at that time the Italian Study Group of Paediatric Radiology.

He was also amongst the first to establish contacts with other paediatric radiologists outside Italy. Furthermore, he was the leading person amongst a small group of Italian paediatric radiologists that consisted of G. Garibaldi, P. Gugliantini, G. Iannaccone (Rome), G.S. Marchese (Turin), N. Macarini, A. Pelizza (Genoa), R. Pinto (Naples), and E. Schiavetti (Milan), who attended the First *Réunion Internationale de Radiologie Pédiatrique* held in Paris in May, 1963. In so doing, they became founding members of the ESPR.

In the following years, he encouraged further colleagues (G.F. Vichi, F. Bellini, G. Golfieri, S. Fasanelli, P.G. Franceschini) to attend the meetings of the newly formed ESPR. He organized the first Italian Symposium of Paediatric Radiology, which was held in Turin on the 13th of October,

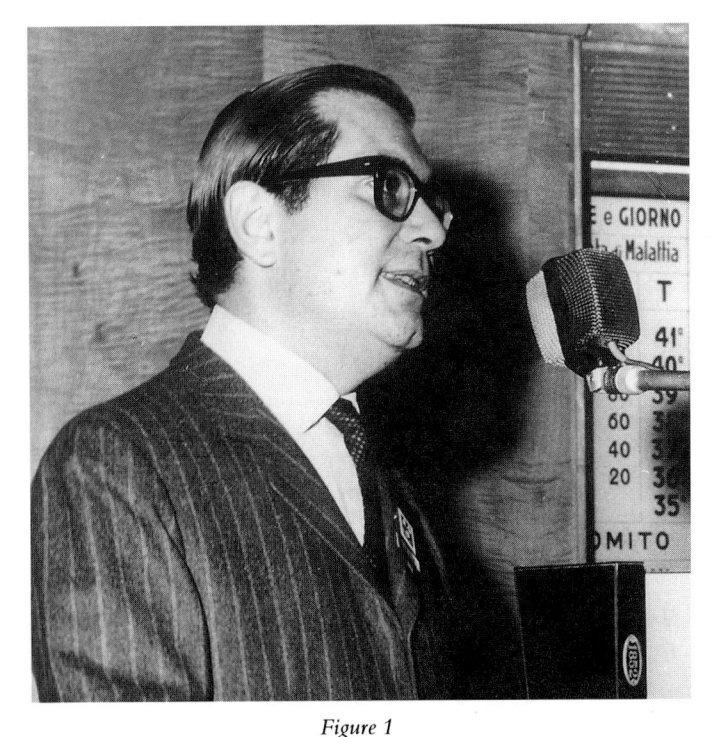

Figure 1
G. S. Marchese, speaking during the opening ceremony of the "First Italian Symposium of Paediatric Radiology" (Turin, 13th October 1968)

1968 (Fig. 2). He also made possible the first refresher course in paediatric radiology ever held in Italy, which took place during the 24th Congress of the Italian Society of Radiology and Nuclear Medicine (SIRMN), held in Palermo in April, 1970.

In addition, he wrote the only treatise on general paediatric radiology ever published in this country (Marchese 1971). In this large book of two volumes, he arranged for the neuroradiology section to be written by A. J. Raimondi, and in so doing recognized the importance of international cooperation in our field.

The untimely death of Marchese on March 17, 1970, left a great void, not only in his department (his successor was M. Randaccio), but in the whole sphere of Italian paediatric radiology. This also explains the lack of national and international symposia in Italy at this time.

Apart from the organization of the Seventh Annual Meeting of the ESPR in Rome (April 16–18, 1970; Figs. 3, 4) which was under the presi-

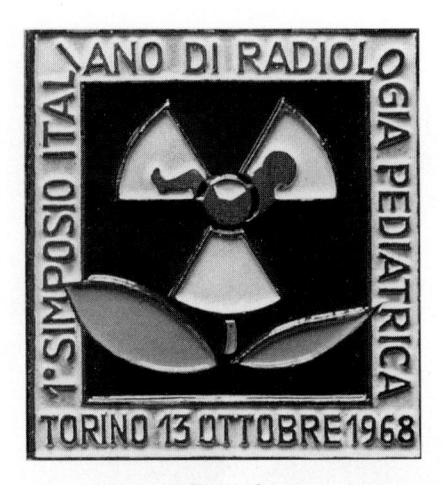

Figure 2
Badge given to the attendants of the "First Italian Symposium of Paediatric Radiology" held
in Turin on the 13th October 1968

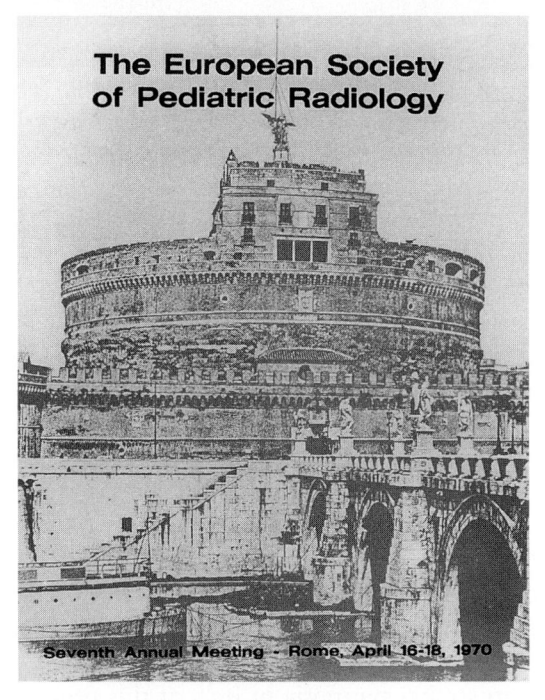

Figure 3
Front cover of the book of abstracts of the seventh Annual Meeting of the ESPR held in
Rome (16th–18th April 1970)

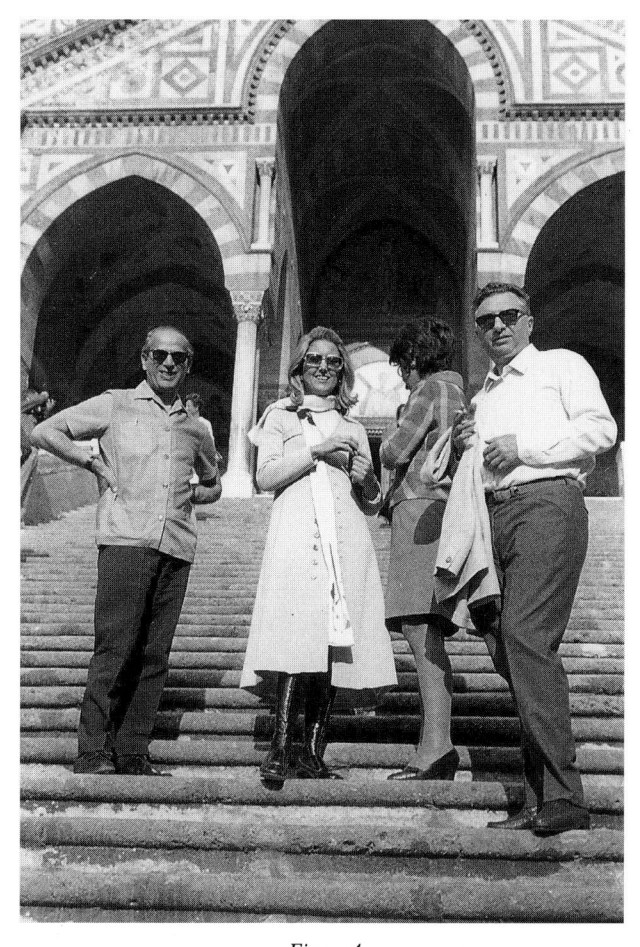

Figure 4
A pleasant moment during the post-congress tour of the Seventh Annual Meeting. S. P. Rawson, Mrs. M. Fasanelli, Mrs. M. L. Iannaccone and G. Iannaccone on the steps of the cathedral at Amalfi

dency of G. Iannaccone (bravely assisted by the young S. Fasanelli and all paediatric radiologists in Rom), there were no further national meetings of Italian paediatric radiology at that time.

Indeed, it was not until C. Sandomenico organized the First National Meeting of the Study Group of Paediatric Radiology of the SIRMN in Naples (11th May 1974; Fig. 5), and A. Pelizza organized the Second National Meeting of Paediatric Radiology in Genoa (27–28 September,

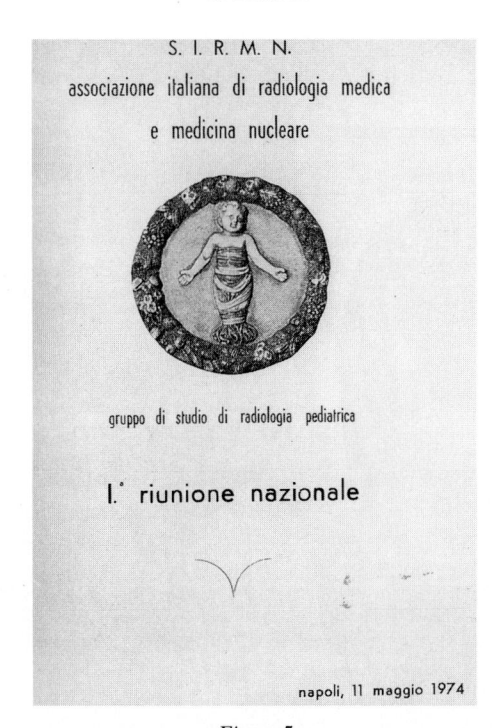

Figure 5
Front cover of the book of abstracts of the "First National Meeting of the Study Group of Paediatric Radiology of the SIRMN" held in Naples (11th of May, 1974)

1975) that the section of Paediatric Radiology of the SIRMN was founded (Fig. 6). During the latter meeting it received an official "blessing" by Prof. L. Oliva on behalf of the SIRMN, and by Prof. J. Sauvegrain on behalf of the ESPR.

This group meets annually, either by holding its own separate congress or by conducting its own sessions during the National Congress of the Italian Society of Radiology (now SIRM), the latter being held every second year.

During the 1960s, new sections of paediatric radiology were opened, namely in Padua, Pavia, Parma and Modena. Those who were involved in the development of these sections are now in their late forties/early fifties and can be considered to be the third generation of paediatric radiologists in Italy. Their training was not only self-initiated, but occurred in different departments of paediatric radiology around the country, and also abroad.

Overseas training was undertaken by T. M. Gajno in Chicago at the Children's Hospital and Cook County Children's Hospital (from 1968 to 1970); G. Beluffi in Birmingham under the guidance of R. Astley (1972) and in Boston for short periods with Prof. J. A. Kirkpatrick (1983 and 1985); R. Perale in Heidelberg with Prof. H. Willich (1975) and in Paris with Prof. C. Fauré (1980); G. Perri in Cape Town with Prof. B. Cremin (1976); P. Toma' in Paris with Prof. C. Fauré (1978); M. Randaccio in Boston (1978 and 1982) and in New York at the Presbyterian Hospital (1981); C. Carini in Paris with Prof. C. Fauré (1981) and in Rochester (MN) at the Mayo Clinics with Prof. A. Hoffmann (1984); L. Artesani in Paris with Prof. J. Sauvegrain (1982); R. Jenuso in Paris with Dr. P. Chaumont and Dr. J. Bennet (1983) and with Prof. C. Fauré (1984); E. Carnevale in Boston with Prof. J. A. Kirkpatrick (1986); and A. Taccone in Toronto with Prof. D. Harwood-Nash (1986).

The appreciation expressed abroad of the work being done by these "old", "middle-aged", and "young" paediatric radiologists was recognized by the ESPR, such that in 1984 (April 11–14), Florence was chosen as the location of the 21st congress of the Society (under the presidency of Dr. G. F. Vichi).

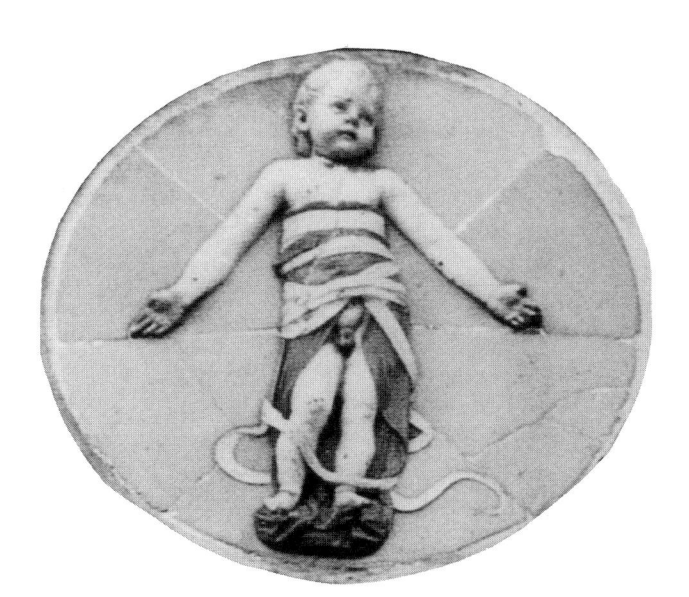

Figure 6
Della Robbia's tondo, on the façade of the *Spedale degli Innocenti* in Florence, is the symbol of paediatric radiology in Italy

From the above-mentioned details, it must be very clear to the reader that paediatric radiology started in Italy in different towns and initially developed locally. Subsequently, general radiologists who had no official training in paediatric radiology (really self-made paediatric radiologists) contributed to the field.

Very rarely, however, brief training abroad was undertaken by some. Maria Pellini is the only person who, to my knowledge, received training abroad at the *Kinderspital* in Zurich in the mid-1930s, and this appears to have been the start of paediatric radiology in Italy. Then it was not until the late 1950s that G. Iannaccone spent 1 year (1958) at the Children's Hospital Medical Center in Boston, where he trained under the guidance of E. D. B. Neuhauser.

From the 1950s onwards, young specialists in radiology also trained in paediatric radiology and usually obtained a position in teaching hospitals. This happened to a greater extent in Genoa, Milan, Turin and Rome.

It must be stressed "ad nauseam" that the formation of the ESPR has had a great impact on the development of paediatric radiology in this country. It not only enabled the independently working radiologists to meet and get to know each other; it also encouraged the understanding of local and general problems and made possible the exchange of vital information between themselves and with their European and American colleagues. This helped to change thinking patterns, not only those of paediatric radiologists about their work in general, but also those of many colleagues (especially paediatricians) about paediatric radiology.

By the middle of the 1960s, paediatric radiology had become a true field of research, study and development, through which a lot could be done for the welfare of patients, especially since it had become so relatively easy to exchange information about equipment (the cumbersome and dangerous machines of the early days were made obsolete by improved technology), research and all the tricks of the trade. It was at this time that significant contributions to the literature of paediatric radiology were made, not only via oral contributions at the meetings of the ESPR (Macarini and Romano 1963, Marchese 1963, Pelizza et al. 1963, Schiavetti 1963, Pelizza and Gemme 1964, Vichi 1965, Pelizza 1967, Pinto et al. 1967, Bellini and Masera 1967, Golfieri et al. 1967, Gajno and Raimondi 1970, Sandomenico and Cerasuolo 1970) and published papers (Iannaccone et al. 1965, Iannaccone 1966, Marchese et al. 1966, Marchese et al. 1968, Galluzzi and De Filippi 1968, Gugliantini 1969, Marchese 1969, Iannaccone and Capotorti 1969, Franceschini et al. 1970, Franceschini et al. 1971, Vichi and Pampaloni 1971), but also via monographs (Cesarini and Gugliantini 1963, Nori Bufalini and Vichi 1966, Barbaccia and Bellini 1968).

As paediatricians were the primary beneficiaries of this new field, they immediately realized how important paediatric radiology was, and how much more important it could become. This was also very well understood (there is always a dark side of the story) by the academic world of radiology which, fearing new dichotomies (as in the very traumatic and never forgotten field of neuroradiology), made all academic positions completely inaccessible to paediatric radiologists. Thus, paediatric radiologists in Italy have lived and still are living in a kind of limbo between general radiology and university hospitals. This is why in Italy there is no professor of Paediatric Radiology. All of us working in sections or departments of paediatric radiology within a university hospital are at the most, *"professore a contratto"* (perhaps similar to honorary senior lecturers) in paediatric radiology.

Official opinion would have us believe that for the SIRM, paediatric radiology is (or was in the late 1970s/early 1980s) one of its most promising branches. Indeed, the ties with SIRN are satisfactory, but there are few practical results in terms of official positions in hospitals (apart from those available in the hospitals listed above) and universities. Within the Executive Committee of the SIRM, none of the presidents of the various branches of radiology are officially represented. This fact applies to paediatric radiology as well. Nevertheless, the needs, hopes, and suggestions of each branch of radiology can be brought to the Committee through one of the committee members, who is officially in charge of this type of liaison.

The ties with the National Society of Paediatrics are good, but they have been better. Paediatric radiologists are very often requested to attend paediatric meetings in order to present the results of their studies. These reports or "lessons" are usually very much appreciated.

Unfortunately for us, paediatricians have not been able to convince general radiologists that paediatric radiologists need more room (academically speaking), nor have they been able to ask for special positions in paediatric radiology through the Board of Professors of Paediatrics in the National Council of Universities.

Due to all of the above circumstances, a few straightforward practical consequences result. The positions available are rare, and so, "sic stantibus rebus", few people want to be trained in this field that, no matter how fascinating it might be, is not financially nor academically satisfactory. This is especially true in these days of high-cost technology (MRI, CT and so on), when very few departments of paediatric radiology can afford the cost. Thus, for all other departments the future appears dim. On a wider scale, the outlook is gloomy. The fate of paediatric radiology in general ultimately depends on general radiology units, where these expensive procedures must be performed and interpreted. The number of full-time paediatric radiologists probably is between 70 and 80 in the whole of Italy, but this figure may be an overestimation. The number of those in specific training in paediatric radiology is very small (not more than 10–15), but a good many trainees in general radiology do receive some training in general paediatric radiology; this varies in extent, however, from one School of Radiology to another.

The list of retired paediatric radiologists is a short one, consisting of P. Gugliantini, C. Sandomenico, M. Randaccio, C. Montanelli, A. Lucchi.

Acknowledgements. I am very much indebted to all of my colleagues who helped me in this research, but most of all to G. De Filippi, G. Iannaccone, C. Montanelli, A. Pelizza, E. Schiavetti, and G. F. Vichi.

References

Barbaccia F, Bellini F (1968) Diagnostica radiologica dell'apparato respiratorio nel primo anno di vita. Casa Editrice Ambrosiana, Milan

Bellini F, Masera G (1967) Les altérations du squelette dans la thalassémie: des variétés et des modifications en rapport à la thérapie transfusionelle. In: Book of Abstracts, Fourth Annual Meeting of the ESPR, Basel, April 13–15, p 53

Bompiani C (1957) I tumori renali dell'eta' pediatrica. Nuntius Radiol 23:529–569

Bulgarelli R, De Maestri A (1952–1953) Ricerche angiopneumografiche nella patologia respiratoria infantile. Ann Radiol Diagnos 25:125–148

Cesarini M, Gugliantini P (1963) Diagnostica radiologica delle malformazioni congenite dell'apparato digerente. SEU – Societa' Editrice Universo, Rome

De Giuli G (1954) Le manifestazioni radiologiche di ostruzione bronchiale in corso di tubercolosi primaria. Radiol Med 40:625–637

Franceschini P, Marchese GS, Fabris C, Ponzone A (1970) Le nanisme tanatophore dans le cadre des nanismes pseudo-achondroplasiques. Ann Radiol 13:399–404

Franceschini P, Grassi E, Marchese GS (1971) Les principaux signes radiologiques du syndrome 4p-. Ann Radiol 14:335–340

Gajno T, Raimondi AJ (1970) Angiographic diagnosis of Arnold-Chiari malformation in the newborn. In: Book of Abstracts, Seventh Annual Meeting of the ESPR, Rome, April 16–18, p 12

Galluzzi W, De Filippi G (1968) Il ruolo della radiologia nello studio del reflusso vescicoureterale dell'-eta' pediatrica. Min Radiol 13:401–407

Golfieri G, Vianello A, Buzzi F, Aluigi A (1967) La dysplasie congénitale de la hanche chez le nouveau-né: diagnostic et prophylaxie thérapeutique. In: Book of Abstracts, Fourth Annual Meeting of the ESPR, Basel, April 13–15, p 1

Gugliantini P (1969) Pseudotumori del torace e dell' addome nell'infanzia. Riv Radiol 9:625–643 (presented at the Sixth Annual Meeting of the ESPR, Warsaw, May 22–24, 1969)

Iannaccone G, Bucci G, Savignoni PG (1965) Diagnostic and prognostic value of X-ray findings in respiratory distress syndrome of newborn premature infants. Ann Radiol 8:237–244

Iannaccone G (1966) Ureteral reflux in normal infants. Ann Radiol 9:31–36
Iannaccone G, Capotorti L (1969) Contribution au syndrome dit "Pseudo-Hurler". Observation de deux sœurs avec des altérations osseuses particulièrement sévères. Ann Radiol 12:355–364
Lischi G, Menichini G (1959) Röntgencraniologia infantile. Edizioni Minerva Medica, Turin
Macarini N, Romano C (1963) Aspects radiologiques des poumons dans la mucoviscidose. In: Book of Abstracts, Réunion Internationale de Radiologie Pédiatrique, Paris, May 2–4, p 44
Marchese GS (1963) La radiologie du prématuré: problèmes techniques et diagnostic. In: Book of Abstracts, Réunion Internationale de Radiologie Pédiatrique, Paris, May 2–4, p 51
Marchese GS, Bono G, Madon E, Grassi E (1966) Importance de l'examen téléradiographie standard dans l'interprétation de l'evolution des cardiopathies congénitales (cardiopathies non cyanogènes). (Examen critique de 657 cases). Ann Radiol 9:85–98
Marchese GS, Albini G, Balocco A, Grasi E (1968) Etude statistique des mensurations angulaires et linéaires de la cavité cotyloïdienne pour le pronostic des dysplasies de la hanche sans luxation. Ann Radiol 11:267–275
Marchese GS (1969) Les causes rares d'obstruction du tube digestif chez le nourrisson et chez l'enfant. Ann Radiol 12:181–190
Marchese GS (1971) Radiologia Pediatrica. Edizioni Minerva Medica, Turin
Nori Bufalini G, Vichi GF (1966) Il neuroblastoma. Edizioni Minerva Medica, Turin
Pelizza A, Rizzo V, Bertolotti E (1963) Etude radiologique des jumeaux xiphoiléopagus. In: Book of Abstracts, Réunion Internationale de Radiologie Pédiatrique, Paris, May 2–4, p 27
Pelizza A, Gemme G (1964) La radiologie dans les affections intestinale aigues du prématuré. In: Book of Abstracts, Première Session de la Société Européenne de Radiologie Pédiatrique. Paris, May 14–16, p 40
Pelizza A (1967) Arthrographie de la luxation congénitale de la hanche. In: Book of Abstracts, Fourth Annual Meeting of the ESPR, Basel, April 13–15, p 7
Pellini M (1934) Contributo clinico-radiologico allo studio della calcolosi vescicale nei bambini. La Pediatria 1:1–23
Pellini M (1940) Sulla ipertrofia del timo. Contributo clinico e radiologico di novanta casi. Clin Ped 22:1–149
Pinto R, Monteleone V, Iannelli L (1967) Valeur des angles du toit acétabulique et du bout supérieur du fémur en rapport aux techniques thérapeutiques employées. In: Book of Abstracts, Fourth Annual Meeting of the ESPR, Basel, April 13–15, p 5
Sandomenico C, Cerasuolo F (1970) Hypophosphatasia in the newborn. In: Book of Abstracts, Seventh Annual Meeting of the ESPR, Rome, April 16–18, p 11
Schiavetti E (1963) Aspects radiographiques des métastases osseuses des sympathoblastomes. In: Book of Abstracts, Réunion Internationale de Radiologie Pédiatrique, Paris, May 2–4, p 25
Vichi GF (1965) Problèmes de technique et de diagnostic de l'occlusion intestinale due à volvulus chez le nouveau-né. In: Book of Abstracts, Second Annual Meeting of the ESPR, Stockholm, May 20–22, p 27
Vichi GF, Pampaloni A (1971) La sialographie dans les affections inflammatoires et néoplasiques des glandes salivaires de l'enfant. Ann Radiol 14:481–490

Paediatric Radiology in the Netherlands

P. P. G. KRAMER

The Pre-ESPR Period

As far as we know, the first medical X-ray in the Netherlands was made on January 28th, 1896, exactly 1 month after the announcement of Röntgen's discovery of the X-ray (Hofmann 1896; Hart 1988). Even after an exposure time of 75 min the structure of the hand is not clearly visible enough to determine the skeletal age of the "patient", but we know that it was a young lady of 22 years, daughter of the director (M.D.) of a medical institution. This experiment was described in a brochure of a secondary school in Maastricht (Hofmann 1896). It was the first publication in the Netherlands on radiology. The first certain paediatric X-ray was made at March 12, 1896. It shows the hand of a 10- to 11-year-old child after an exposure time of 1 h and 18 min. The X-ray was made in the same laboratory as the above-mentioned picture (Fig. 1).

In September 1908, the 4th International Congress on Electrology and Radiology was held in Amsterdam. Scheltema, a paediatrician, presented the first known Dutch paper about the use of radiology in children, entitled "Die Permeation und die Röntgendiagnostik bei der Untersuchung des Magendarmkanales". Scheltema used a fluoroscope in children to follow an intestinal catheter with an opaque end and localize the tip. He was able to aspirate fluid or place drugs at the correct place into the small bowel without being influenced by the stomach acid (Wylick 1966). At that time there were six paediatric hospitals in the Netherlands. Four of them still exist. All are named after a member (mostly a queen) of the royal family: The *Sophia Kinderziekenhuis* (SKZ) in Rotterdam (since 1863), the *Emma Kinderziekenhuis* (EKZ) in Amsterdam (since 1865), the *Juliana Kinderziekenhuis* (JKZ) in The Hague (since 1885) and the *Wilhelmina Kinderziekenhuis* (WKZ) in Utrecht (since 1888). There were also paediatric hospitals in Arnhem (since 1882) and in Dordrecht (since 1885). The Sophia Children's Hospital in Rotterdam had an X-ray installation as early as 1901

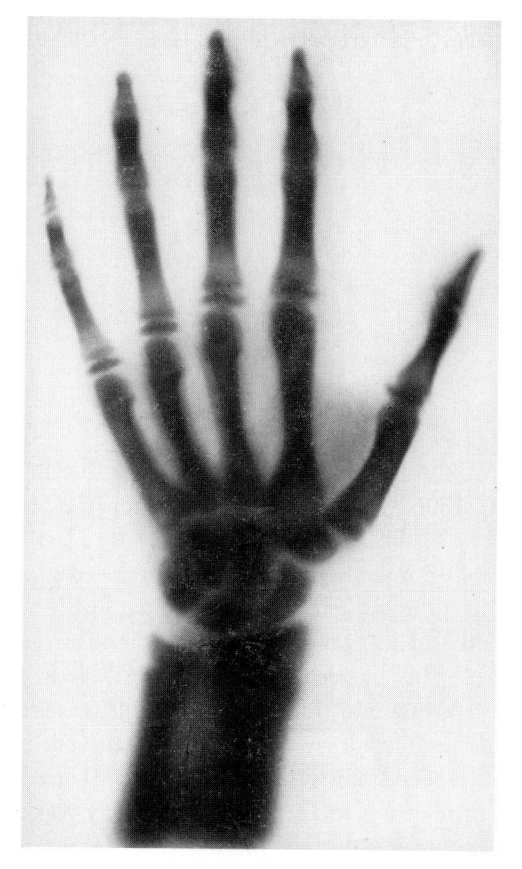

Figure 1
First medical X-ray, of a child's hand, in the Netherlands, March 12, 1896

(Lieburg 1975) and the Wilhelmina Children's Hospital in 1909, which was operated by paediatricians until the beginning of the 1970s. Paediatric radiology in the Netherlands was (and is) also done by general radiologists. Later on, some of them came to the paediatric hospitals to review the pictures made by the paediatricians.

The ESPR Period

Paediatric radiology had its real start only when some specialised paediatric radiologists took their education and training into their own hands (fellowships of some months, or a year abroad). These pioneers were: Allard Botenga (AB), since 1967 in the JKZ; Morteza Meradji (MM), since 1970 in the SKZ; Peter Kramer (PK) since 1973 in the WKZ and Chris Staalman (CS), since 1978 in the EKZ; these full-time paediatric radiologists became members of the ESPR in 1970 (PK), 1974 (MM, CS) and 1975 (AB).

The participation at ESPR congresses started in 1967 with Henk Sanchez, general radiologists from Maastricht, and Dini van Dijk, a well-known initiator for the national and international societies of technicians. From 1971 (PK) and 1972 (MM and CS) on, most of the above-mentioned people regularly attended the ESPR meetings. Allard Botenga joined the congresses in 1974 and Frits Bröker (FB) in 1977. In 1973, these paediatric radiologists formed the "Dutch Group of Paediatric Radiologists" (DGPR), which started to meet three times a year.

The impact of paediatric radiology on the education of general radiologists increased in the years that followed. As a stimulus, the ESPR decided to have a meeting in the Netherlands in 1980, organized by the DGPR. Because the ESPR decided to assign the congress to a country instead of to a person, the annotation of this congress in congress books is always made in this way.

Because of its scientific niveau (MM), its location at the beach in Scheveningen, and its perfect social program, this congress was a great success. It certainly had a positive effect on the status of paediatric radiology in the Netherlands. Paediatric radiology became more and more a part of the curriculum for general radiologists, and now it is obligatory, with a separate examination. The ties with the Dutch Society for Radiodiagnostics are strong. Postgraduate courses are organized by DGPR with Peter Kramer as co-ordinator. This resulted in the first book in Dutch on paediatric radiology (editor PK). Many courses for paediatricians and technicians on paediatric radiology were organized. The DGPR has grown with the addition of Albert Martijn (AM), Paediatric Radiologist at the University Hospital of Groningen since 1983 (ESPR member since 1986), Simon Robben (SR), paediatric radiologist at the *Sophia Kinderziekenhuis* in Rotterdam since 1987, and Erik Beek (EB), paediatric radiologist in the *Wilhelmina Kinderziekenhuis* at Utrecht since 1989. The last two will become ESPR members in 1992. The first full-time professor in paediatric radiology is Morteza Meradji (1991).

The DGPR consists now of seven full-time paediatric radiologists (MM, CS, AB, AM, SR, EB, PK), four part-time paediatric radiologists – Frits Bröker (Apeldoorn), C. Hitge-Boetes (Nijmegen), N. M. Zonderland (The Hague) and T. Prins (Groningen) – and about 20 interested general radiologists. They all meet three times a year, alternating between Utrecht and another hospital.

During the 20 years of Dutch participation in ESPR congresses many papers and posters have been submitted and presented. Besides the organization of the ESPR meeting in Scheveningen, Dutch Radiologists have participated on the board of the ESPR. One was a member of the nominating commity (CS), one a member of the board during the Congress of 1980 (AB), and one is president – elect for 1995 (PK).

During the congresses, in addition to active participation through presentation of papers and posters, some Dutch participants were members of the Scientific Committee (MM, PK), and moderators. One is a member of the Lake Starnberg Group (PK).

Although paediatric radiology in the Netherlands is practised by only seven full-time paediatric radiologists, their impact is growing. Besides the children's hospitals, there are eight university hospitals in the Netherlands. Of the four original paediatric hospitals, one (EKZ) has joined the general university hospital in Amsterdam, and the JKZ will soon be part of a general hospital. In the near future there will be only two relatively large children's hospitals, one in Rotterdam (SKZ, 1993) and one in Utrecht (WKZ, 1998). Each hospital will have 200–220 beds. Among the remaining university hospitals there is a full-time paediatric radiologists at the Amsterdam Medical Centre [with the EKZ (CS)] and at the University Hospital of Groningen (AM). The University Hospital of Nijmegen has a part-time paediatric radiologist (C. H. B. Hitge-Boetes), the University Hospital of Leiden has no paediatric radiologists but is affiliated with the *Juliana Kinderziekenhuis*. The hospital of the Free University (V. U.) of Amsterdam and the University Hospital of Maastricht have no paediatric radiologists. However, even in these hospitals without a paediatric radiologist, general radiologists with an interest in paediatric radiology have begun to put the field on a higher level. Because of the few positions available for paediatric radiologists it is not worthwhile to start a training programme in paediatric radiology in the Netherlands. Radiologists who are interested in working full- or part-time in paediatric radiology are advised to obtain an education in one of the remaining paediatric hospitals and to apply for fellowhips outside the Netherlands. The quality and the level of paediatric radiology in the children's hospitals and in those hospitals with a paediatric radiologist is comparable to that of well-known paediatric radiology centres elsewhere.

Because of the relatively small dimension of the paediatric hospitals, it is very difficult to provide all the imaging modalities and there has to be a compromise. There should be close cooperation between the university hospitals and the children's hospitals, to ensure that examinations of children conform to the standards for paediatric radiology. Timing and equipment should be adapted to children's needs. Technicians with good training in paediatric radiology and paediatric radiologists should be in charge of the examinations.

The ESPR has been of great help in developing paediatric radiology in the Netherlands. Not only on the board but also amongst the individual members of the Society we all have many good friends.

Most members of the DGPR became ESPR members in a period when we regarded congresses as family reunions rather than as ESPR meetings. This gives an idea of the atmosphere amongst its members. Without the help of all these friends paediatric radiology in the Netherlands would not have grown as it has. We hope the ESPR will have a long, continuously successful future and we all hope to participate at the annual meetings for many years to come. For the friendship that we have experienced from various members of the society we thank them all very much.

References

Hart PD 't (1988) Het zieke kind in goede handen, uitgever. Catema, Zwolle
Hofmann HJ (1896) Proefnemeningen met de röntgensche strahlen, uitgever. Leiter-Nijpels, Maastricht
Lieburg MJ van (1975) Het Sophia Kinderziekenhuis 1863–1975. Rotterdam
Wylick WAH van (1966) Uitgever. Hoeijenbos, Utrecht

Pediatric Radiology in Poland*

A. Marciński

In Warsaw, on February 18, 1896, the physicist Wiktor Biernacki delivered a lecture on X-rays, and on May 19 of the same year, Mikołaj Brunner, head physician of the Holy Ghost Hospital, at a meeting of the Warsaw Medical Society, demonstrated 20 roentgenograms made by means of a personally constructed apparatus (Fig. 1). In the same year, Brunner published an article in the *Medical Gazette* entitled "Roentgen rays and roentgenography and their medical applications".

In Poland before the discovery of roentgen rays, pediatrics was in its beginnings. The first pediatric clinic, opened in Cracow in 1874 and headed by Prof. Maciej Jakubowski, a renowned educator of pediatricians, was not prepared in its modest circumstances to introduce radiodiagnosis in diseases of children. In spite of the primitive character of the early sources of roentgen rays, radiodiagnosis was applied first in surgery, and then in internal medicine, before it was used in pediatrics.

Nonetheless, the possibilities inherent in the rays discovered by Roentgen aroused the interest of pediatricians. The first mention of their use in pediatrics may be found in the memoirs of the Therapeutic Department for Children at Ogrodowa Street in Warsaw, which existed from 1893 to 1911. In 1912, Bączkiewicz, head physician of the hospital, wrote: "As soon as a roentgen laboratory was opened at the neighboring Holy Ghost Hospital, we applied to its head for permission to make use of it for the examination of poor children without cost. That permission was granted on May 24, 1901." Although nothing is known of the scope of the examinations, undoubtedly they pertained mainly to the skeletal system. The experience thus gained prompted Bączkiewicz to propose installation of roentgen units in children's hospitals. Upon receiving a donation of 3000 rubles (his own hospital being in the course of liquidation), Bączkiewicz in 1911

---

* This article is based on the paper by A. K. Rowiński and A. Marciński (1972) Beginnings and development of pediatric radiology in Poland. *Polish Review of Radiology and Nuclear Medicine* 36:135–142.

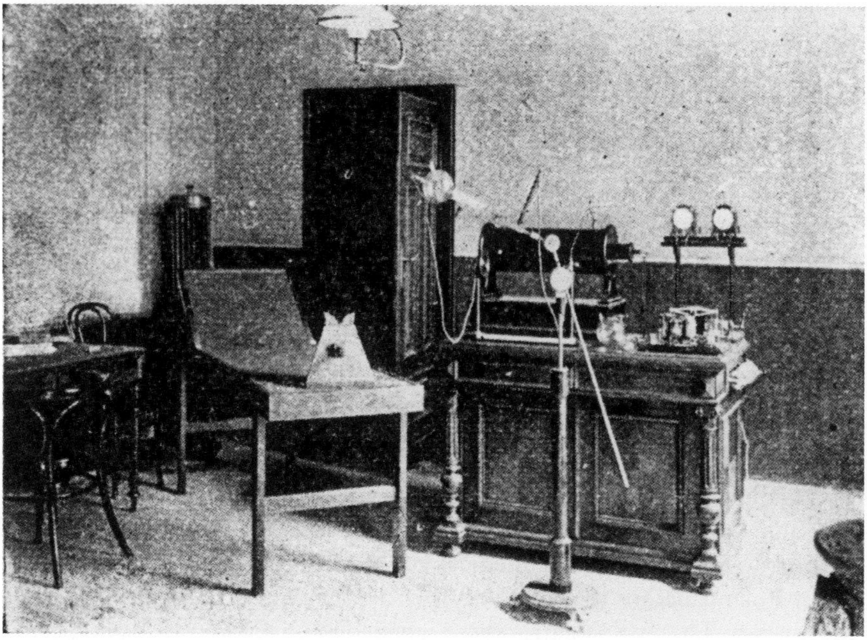

Figure 1
First X-ray room in Warsaw (1896) at Holy Ghost Hospital

placed this sum at the disposal of the Warsaw Hospital for Children at Kopernik Street "for the specific purpose of financing the roentgen laboratory."

The Warsaw Hospital for Children, the first pediatric hospital in Warsaw (and second in Poland after St. Sophie Hospital in Lwów) was founded in 1869 by Antoni Sikorski, but it did not receive a roentgen unit until 1914. On the 100th anniversary of the hospital, in 1969, Wybieralski wrote: "For roentgendiagnosis, the surgical department at first made use of a transportable apparatus borrowed from S. Trojanowski, a Warsaw roentgenologist. In 1933, a small roentgen apparatus, adapted also for radiography of the chest, was installed." Besides Trojanowski, the radiologists Marian Kowalewski and Karol Vincenz were employed at the hospital.

In 1878, 9 years after the Warsaw Hospital for Children, the Berson and Bauman Memorial Hospital was opened. In its report (Poznański 1916) for the period up to 1915, we read: "Roentgen examinations were made voluntarily by Rubinroth without remuneration," and "Bacteriological and roentgenological laboratories are being planned." In the 20-year interwar period, an eminent Warsaw radiologist working at the hospital, Benjamin

Kryński (1934), writing about advances in roentgenology between 1924 and 1934, emphasized that advances in roentgenologic technique "have made possible good roentgenograms of the mobile organs (heart, lungs), especially in children."

Most of the information about roentgen examinations in this period, however, is provided by two reports covering 20 years at the Charles and Mary Hospital in Warsaw, written by W. Szenajch (1924, 1935) its head. This hospital was opened in 1913, and from the beginning it had a roentgen laboratory and chemical and bacteriological laboratories. In the first 10 years (1913–1923), 1181 roentgenograms were made for the surgical department (in which 3231 patients were treated), 288 for the internal diseases department, and 713 for ambulatory patients. In the same 10-year period, 810 fluoroscopies were carried out (Szenajch 1926). Thus, in the years 1913–1923, a total of 2992 roentgen examinations were done, including 2182 films, of which 1523 pertained to diseases and bone traumas. From the report for the second 10-year period (1924–1934) we learn that "the roentgen apparatus, after many years of use, has become worn out." In 1926 a new roentgen apparatus was purchased and, significantly, was installed in quarters next to both the surgical and internal diseases departments. The number of children examined increased from 2992 to 5504 in the second 10-year period. The proportion of films of the internal organs increased somewhat; whereas in the first 10 years 71% of films were of the skeletal system, in the second decade this proportion dropped to 61% (Szenajch 1935).

In 1934, Krystyna Ossowska, a pupil of the eminent radiologist Maria Werkenthin, joined the staff of the hospital. However, the development of the Charles and Mary Hospital and of pediatric radiology was interrupted by the outbreak of World War II. The hospital was entirely demolished, and after the war the surviving physicians organized a new hospital at the site of the present Clinical Hospital of the Medical Academy at 3, Działdowska Street.

Let us now look at the development of pediatric radiology in the early period in other parts of Poland.

In the 19th century a children's hospital was opened in Poznań (the present Provincial Children's Hospital). Although the hospital existed from 1877, it did not have a roentgenologic laboratory until 1924/1925.

The first modern children's hospital in Poland, the Anna Marie Hospital in Łódź, opened in 1905 by Józef Brudziński, was equipped like western European hospitals. In 1908 a roentgen apparatus was installed, which, according to a report of the head physician T. Mogilnicki 1930, was replaced in 1927, after being used for 20 years, by a small diagnostic roentgen apparatus. According to the hospital report for 1929 (the hospital then had 180 beds), 691 children were examined, including 604 fluoroscopies and 407 radiographies. Most of the fluoroscopies concerned the chest, and films were taken mainly of the skeletal system.

In Lublin in 1912, Władysław Jasiński, head of the Hospital for Children, wrote in the Second Annual Report of the Hospital: "In view of the fact that pediatric surgery consists largely of orthopedics and mechanotherapy, organization of an Orthopedic Institute possessing a roentgen department should be envisaged." Dr. Jasiński seems to have fully realized the importance of roentgenologic examinations.

In the light of what has been said, it would seem that the Warsaw center was the main cradle of pediatric radiology in Poland.

A new era in the development of pediatric radiology in Poland began in 1925 with the founding of the Polish Radiological Society and in 1926 publication of the *Polish Radiological Review* as its organ. The editorial committee included Zygmunt Stankiewicz, radiologist at the Charles and Mary Pediatric Hospital in Warsaw, and Emil Głowacki, radiologist of the Clinic of Children's Diseases of the Medical Academy in Warsaw. However, the first case report on pediatric radiology was published by Kramsztyk in 1908, on the diagnosis of Barlow's disease.

At first, only the Warsaw branch of the Polish Radiological Society was organized. Already at some of its first meetings problems of pediatric radiology were discussed. In 1925, Adelfang presented a case of "osteitis deformans in a 7-year-old child," and in 1926, Stankiewicz "Multiple cartilaginous exostoses." Shortly thereafter, in 1927, Głowacki reported on a "personal modification of a protected table for radiography in children" and an "orthodiagnostic focusing device," showing that orthodiagrams of the heart were being done at that time at the Children's Clinic of the Warsaw University. In 1927, Głowacki also published a paper on "so-called atypical cases of achondroplasia," and Stankiewicz reported in 1927 about "Osgood-Schlatter disease." Thus, pediatric radiology was beginning to assert itself in Warsaw.

In 1932, upon the initiative of the Polish Radiological Society, the first theoretical and practical course in medical radiology was organized, at which Kryński lectured on pediatric radiology, having considerable experience in that field, especially in the pathology of the respiratory system in children. Space does not allow mention of all the demonstrations and papers on pediatric radiology which became more and more numerous, and with a broader scope than just case reporting. At the meeting of the Polish Radiological Society in Poznan in 1933, B. Kryński spoke on "Intussusception of the small and large intestines in children." At the next convention in Warsaw in 1934, Kryński presented a paper on the "picture of the lungs in whooping cough," and Głowacki and Wiszniewski discussed "tuberculous cavities of the lungs in infants." In 1937, at the second course on medical radiology, Kryński again lectured on roentgendiagnosis in diseases of childhood, and Dr. Stankiewicz and Kowalewski discussed their experience with encephalography and ventriculography. The journals *Polish Surgical Review* and *Medical Journal* published papers on pediatric gastrology and urology. The scope of pediatric radiology began to expand; this is also shown by the first Polish textbook of pediatrics, edited by W. Jasiński in 1938.

Presumably, if the war had not broken out, we might have had a considerable literature in this field, in the form of monographs and textbooks. However, the war interrupted the development of pediatric radiology in our country for 6 long years.

The development of pediatric radiology in Poland after World War II was conected mostly with Warsaw, where Prof. Ksawery Rowiński established the first Chair of Pediatric Radiology in Poland at the Medical Academy (Fig. 2). Beginning in 1976 it was managed by Prof. Andrzej Marciński. Also in the Institute for Mother and Child in Warsaw a Department of Pediatric Radiology and Radiotherapy was formed with Prof. Stanisław Kubicz as head until 1976; it was later managed by Prof. Stefan Winnicki. For many years these two centers were the leading institutions in diagnostics of cardiovascular diseases, respiratory tract diseases, and malignant pediatric pathology.

The next pediatric X-ray laboratory was created by Prof. Kazimierz Pietroń in Lublin in 1955. It later assumed a new shape as the Department of Pediatric Radiology at the Institute of Pediatrics. It has been managed by Prof. K. Pietroń up to the present.

As mentioned, the X-ray Laboratory at the Clinic of Pediatric Diseases of Jagielonski University at Strzelecka Street in Kraków was established in the years 1928–1929. It continued its activity after World War II. However, the actual development of pediatric radiology started only after 1966, with the formation of the Department of Roentgenology at the Pediatric Institute of the Medical Academy in Prokocim. The head of the Department was Kazimierz Kozłowski, later B. Sikorska.

Following World War II in Poznań, the Children's Hospital Department of Roentgenology was developed fully after Maria Solawa took over the management in 1955. Subsequently, a Department of Pediatric Radiology was established in 1971 at the newly formed Institute of Pediatrics at Szpitalna Street. Up to that time, K. Kozłowski was one of the pediatricians

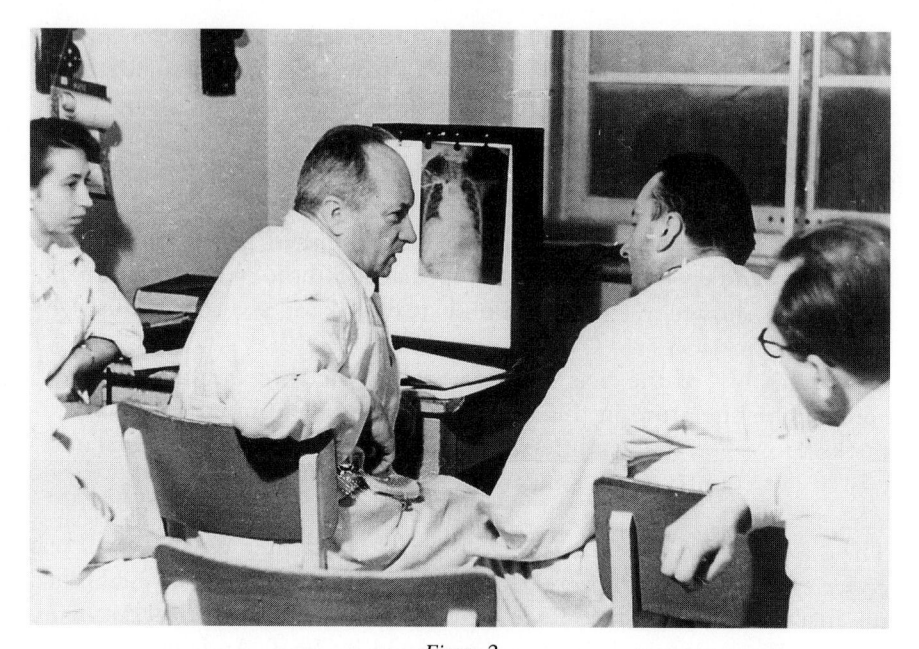

Figure 2
H. Urbanik, Prof. K. Rowiński, A. Chorścicki (*left* to *right*) during a consultation at the Department of Pediatric Radiology in Warsaw, 1957

involved with roentgen diagnostics of the patients treated at the Clinics of Pediatric Diseases of the Medical Academy. In the 1970s the Department of Pediatric Radiology, as part of the Radiology Institute of the Medical Academy, became the leading radiologic center in the Poznań region.

Thus, at the beginning of 1969 Prof. K. Rowiński, Prof. S. Kubicz, A. Jakubowski, B. Słoma-Wałejko, H. Urbanik, D. Kaniewska (Warsaw), K. Kozłowski (Poznań, later Kraków), Sikorska (Kraków), and Prof. K. Pietroń (Lublin) formed the initial team of Polish pediatric radiologists. Around them gathered others who were fascinated by pediatric radiology – the new branch of pediatrics and roentgenology.

There was nothing uncommon about the fact that the radiologists from Poland – Prof. K. Rowiński, Prof. S. Kubicz, A. Jakubowski, K. Kozłowski, and J. Kopczyńska – participated in the International Meeting of Pediatric Radiology in 1963 and at the first Session of the European Society of Pediatric Radiology in Paris in 1964.

The establishment of the European Society of Pediatric Radiology exerted an obvious influence on the development of pediatric radiology in

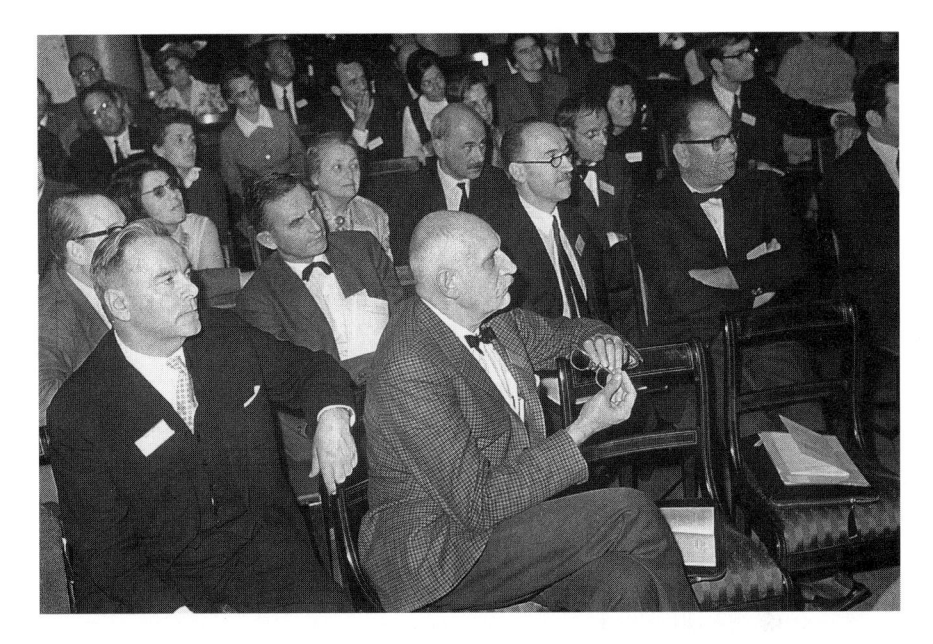

Figure 3
Sixth meeting of the European Society of Pediatric Radiology, Warsaw, 1969. *Left* to *right*: S. Kubicz, D. Prot, J. Lefèbvre, J. Bennet, C. Fauré, J. Sauvegrain, I. Nitz, and H.J. Kaufmann

Poland. Particularly the sixth meeting of the ESPR (Fig. 3–5), which took place in Warsaw in 1969, strengthened the relationship of the pediatric radiologists with the society of general radiologists and pediatricians.

The existence of the ESPR also stimulated the wish of the Polish pediatric radiologists to establish their own society. The Section of Pediatric Radiology of the Polish Medical Radiological Society was created in 1971, the representative of pediatric radiology is a member of the Main Board of our Society. Sessions on pediatric radiology are held at scientific meetings of the Polish Medical Radiological Society.

An academic career is widely open to all pediatric radiologists who are willing to devote the necessary effort. Of 75 members of the Section of Pediatric Radiology, 26 have obtained an M.D. degree. In addition, there are two actively working professors of pediatric radiology: A Marciński in Warsaw and K. Pietrón in Lublin. Professors A. Jakubowski and S. Winnicki, both of Warsaw, have retired.

Unfortunately, several worthy members of radiological society have left us: Prof. K. Rowiński (in 1983), Prof. S. Kubicz (in 1985), B. Ros-

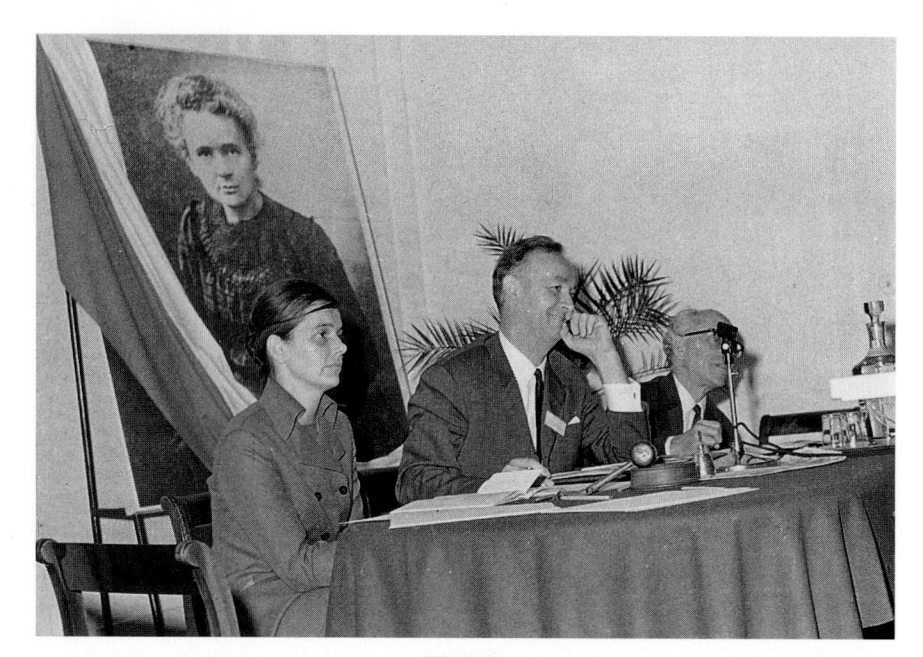

Figure 4
The chair at the ESPR Congress Warsaw in 1969 under the "symbolic aegis" of Madame Curie. Chairman: M. A. Lassrich

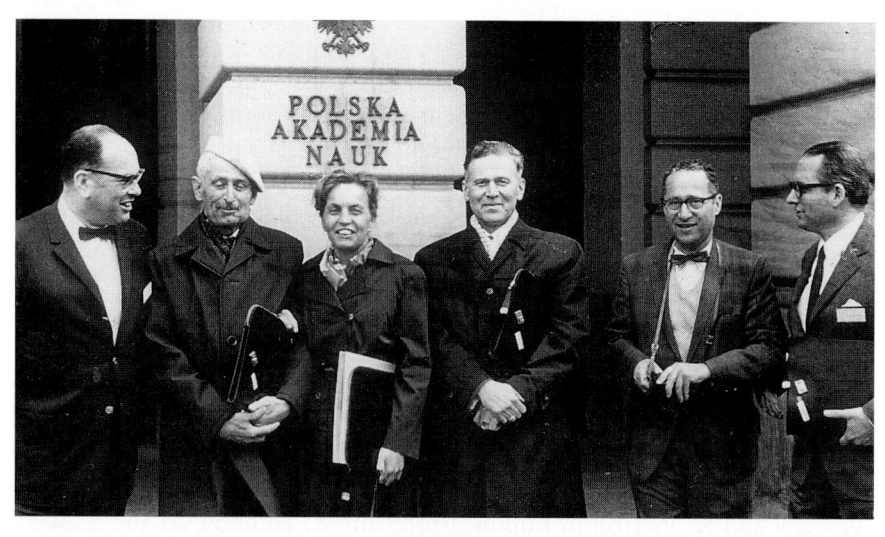

Figure 5
Participants at the ESPR Congress in Warsaw, May 1969. In front of the Polish Academy of Sciences (from the *left*): H. J. Kaufmann, K. Gefferth, Irmgard Greinacher, E. Willich, F. N. Silverman and K. Knapp

nowska (1987), A. Kaniewska (1987), and B. Słoma-Wałejko (1988). However, their knowledge, inquisitiveness, and talents had served to gather around them a sizeable group of students and co-workers for whom the problems of pediatric radiology are still especially important.

References

Bączkiewicz J (1912) Memoirs of the therapeutic ward for children at 17, Ogrodowa street, Warszawa (in Polish)
Biernacki W (1898) New fields of invisible spectrum (in Polish). Warsaw, Biblioteka Dzieł Wyborowych, no 44
Brunner M (1896) Roentgen rays and roentgenography in medicine (in Polish). Gazeta Lekarska 16:28–30
Głowacki E (1927) Personal modification of a protective table for radiography in children (in Polish). Polski Przegląd Radiologiczny 2:39–34
Głowacki E (1927) Orthodiagnostic focusing device (in Polish). Polski Przegląd Radiologiczny 2:140–144
Grudziński Z (1927) So-called atypical forms of achondroplasia (in Polish). Polski Przegląd Radiologiczny 2:106–127
Jasiński W (1912) Second Annual Report of the Children's Hospital in Lublin (in Polish), Lublin
Jasiński W (1936) Diseases of children (in Polish). Ars Medici, Warsaw
Kramsztyk S (1908–1909) On the diagnosis of Barlow's disease (in Polish). Przegląd Pediatryczny 1:136
Kryński B (1934) Last ten years of roentgenology (in Polish). Warszawskie Czasopismo Lekarskie 11:356–358
Mogilnicki T (1930) Twenty-fifth anniversary of the Anna Maria Hospital for Children in Łódź (1905–1930) (in Polish). Łódź
Poznański (1916) Report of the Berson and Bauman Memorial Hospital at Śliska street, Warszawa (1873–1915) (in Polish). Warsaw
Stankiewicz Z (1926) Exostoses cartilagineae multiplices (in Polish). Polski Przegląd Radiologiczny 1:90–93
Stankiewicz Z (1927) Osgood-Schlatter disease (in Polish). Polski Przegląd Radiologiczny 2:281–290
Szenajch W (1926) The Charles and Mary Hospital for Children – first ten years (1913–1923) (in Polish). Warsaw
Szenajch W (1935) The Charles and Mary Hospital for Children – second ten years (1924–1934) (in Polish). Warsaw
Wybieralski A (1969) History of the Warsaw Hospital for Children (1869–1969) (in Polish). PZWL, Warsaw

The History of Pediatric Radiology in Romania

M. RADULESCU

An interest in diagnostic radiology in Romanian hospitals was already recorded in 1896, and in 1897, the first X-ray apparatus was installed at the Military Hospital in Bucharest. Dr Dan Gerota started working with this equipment in 1899. In 1896, several X-ray machines were set up in Iasi through the initiative and effort of Prof. Dr. Hurmusache. By 1925, X-ray equipment was available in some big city hospitals (Brasov, Craiova, Oradea, Sighişoara).

Radiology training was offered in the university hospitals of Bucharest, Iasi and Cluj. Of the Romanian radiology pioneers Prof. Dr. Negru was the most prolific.

Soon after pediatric hospitals were established in the big cities, first pediatric radiology departments were founded. The directors of these departments were actual pediatric radiologists.

Thus, in 1959, at Grigore Alexandrescu Hospital in Bucharest, Dr. Zalman Fruchter succeeded in publishing a wonderful "Atlas of Paediatric Radiology"; this outstanding book, together with "Clinical and Radiological Diagnosis in Paediatrics," written by Dr. Mibai Balaban, working at that time at Bucharest's Mother and Child Care Institute (both early members of the E.S.P.R.) represent the first steps in outlining pediatric radiology as a specialty.

At the same time, between 1955 and 1970, Dr. Victor Rucsa of the Fundeni Hospital in Bucharest, devoted his work completely to pediatric radiology and put together one of the most complete collections of X-ray films.

The personalities already mentioned were followed by other distinguished radiologists: in Bucharest Dr. Liliana Enacheacu (E.S.P.R. member), with special contributions on "Hystiocytosis X Research"; in Cluj Dr. Zoe Nicoara, who has been deeply involved in developing paediatric radiology training, concentrated on respiratory apparatus pathology.

In 1980, when paediatric radiology became accepted as a specialty in its own right, the training of pediatric specialists really started: Dr. Mariana

Radulescu of Maria Sklodowaka Curie Pediatric Hospital in Bucharest; Dr. Goldis Gheorghe of Fundeni Hospital in Bucharest, and Dr. Vlad of the Paediatric Hospital in Iasi.

All these pediatric radiology enthusiasts, with the strong support of Dr. Serban Georgescu, vice-president of the Romanian Radiology Society, succeeded in creating a Pediatric Radiology section within the Romanian Radiology Society in 1990. It is these individuals who are working continuously to further develop this specialty.

Pediatric Radiology in Spain

V. Pérez-Candela and J. Lucaya

In 1962 Professor Suarez, chairman of the Department of Pediatrics at the University Hospital in Seville, established the first pediatric radiology unit in Spain. As head of the department he nominated Klaus Knapp, who had trained in pediatric radiology in Germany with Prevot and Lassrich. Up to that time all radiological examinations in children had been performed by general radiologists. While in Seville, Knapp trained several fellows, including Lanuza, Cortada, and Sánchez Pajares among others.

The Spanish government built two large pediatric hospitals, one in Madrid in 1964 (Hospital La Paz) and the other in Barcelona in 1965 (Hospital Valle de Hebrón). Klaus Knapp and Alvaro Lanuza became the staff pediatric radiologists in the Madrid Hospital, while Antonio Domenech and Santiago Creixell ran the Barcelona facility. In 1970, another pediatric hospital was built in Valencia and Alvaro Lanuza and Victor Pérez-Candela were placed in charge of the pediatric radiology department.

In 1971, Javier Lucaya and Rafael Ramos joined the staff of the Department of Radiology at the Children's Hospital "Valle de Hebrón" in Barcelona. Both had been trained in the USA, Lucaya under Silverman in Cincinnati and Ramos under Kirkpatrick in Philadelphia.

Postgraduate teaching programs in pediatric radiology were developed in all the aforementioned medical centers, where most of the pediatric radiologists currently working in Spain received their training.

In April 1975, Knapp organized the 12th Meeting of the ESPR in Madrid. This meeting permitted some Spanish pediatric radiologists to become acquainted with the European Society and with colleagues from other countries.

In 1983, the Spanish Society of Pediatric Radiology was founded and Victor Pérez-Candela became its first president; he occupied the post until 1988, when it was decided that the presidency should change hands every 2 years. The next president was Antonio Martinez of the Children's Hospital "12 de Octubre" in Madrid, followed in 1990 by Purificación López from the Children's Hospital "Carlos Haya" in Málaga, and in 1992 by Ignacio Pastor of the Children's Hospital "La Paz" in Madrid.

In 1986, the 23rd Meeting of the ESPR was organized in Barcelona by Javier Lucaya. The meeting itself and the preceding postgraduate course enabled a large number of Spanish pediatricians and radiologists to become informed about the state of the art of pediatric radiology.

In 1989, Antonio Martinez organized the first meeting of the Spanish Society of Pediatric Radiology in Madrid. The second meeting, organized by Purificación López, was held in Málaga in 1991. Both were very successful and attracted a large number of participants.

In Spain at present there are 25 children's hospitals and 120 pediatric radiologists who are fighting to have our specialty officially recognized by the Ministry of Health, even though unofficially we are acknowledged to be "radiologists with special dedication to pediatrics."

The History of Pediatric Radiology in Switzerland

A. GIEDION

Introduction

Already in mid-January 1896, Röntgen's discovery, published on January 1st of the same year, was used by Theodor Kocher, the famous Swiss surgeon and later Nobel prize laureate to localize a needle in the hand of one of his patients (Wieser 1989). The date of the first pediatric application of X-rays in Switzerland is unknown. The development of pediatric radiology was intimately connected with the emergence of children's hospitals, established in the second half of the nineteenth century. Originally independent, private, charitable institutions, they eventually became, at least in towns with a medical school, pediatric university centers. Typically, these buildings were situated at sites chosen by the donors because of their "healthy" surrounding, sometimes far away from the major adult hospitals, making later on the joint use of specialized wards and of expensive equipment difficult. This topographical isolation had some influence, positive as well as negative, on the development of pediatric radiology. Furthermore, the federalistic structure of Switzerland, with each canton (state) making health and educational policy largely independent of the federal government, is to some extent responsible for the remarkable difference in the growth of pediatric radiology centers, as will be presented in the subsequent sections of this report. Above all, the interest in radiology of the medical director of the hospital, who usually is also the chairman of pediatrics at the university, and the presence of a "modern" division of pediatric surgery, unable to work properly otherwise, were decisive for the use of this new "tool" and eventually for the acceptance of pediatric radiology as an independent subspecialty. Last but not least, it was due to the personal efforts of three young enthusiastic Swiss pediatricians that pediatric radiology in our country eventually attained an international level. They started their work mostly self-taught in the late 1950s, were further trained and stimulated by fellowships in the USA, France, and Sweden, and were

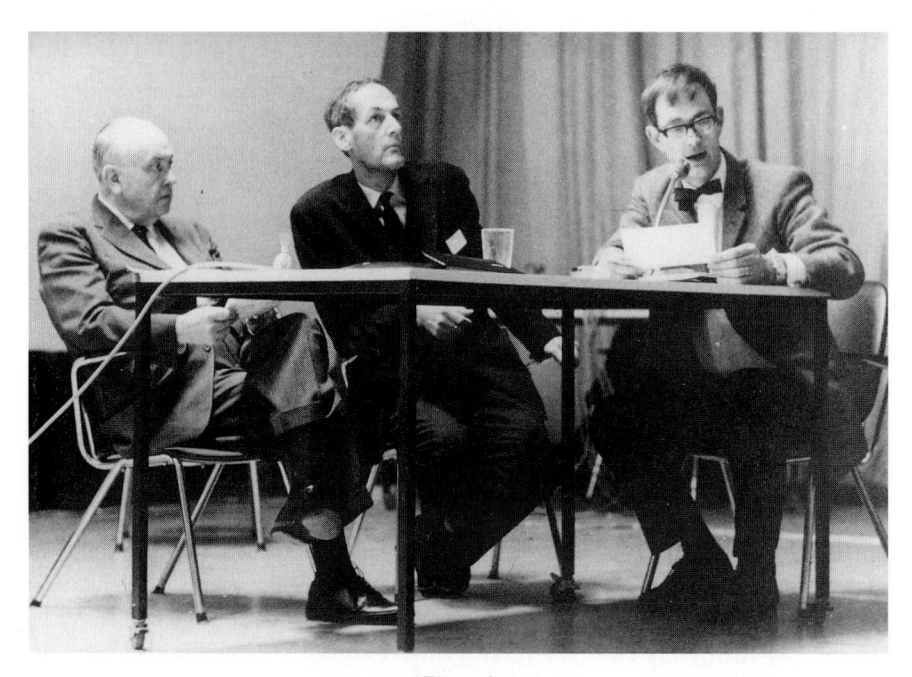

Figure 1
The chair at the Hamburg ESPR meeting in 1968. Dr. Caffey, Dr. Giedion and Dr. Bruns, the secretary of that meeting who was the victim of a car accident 1970

finally supported intellectually and morally by the ESPR, of which they were co-founders. The story of Daniel Nusslé, how he started three Swiss university departments of pediatric radiology (see below) illustrates well this fact. The first X-ray rooms exclusively for children were installed in 1902 and 1904 in Basel and Zürich. The "plates" were exposed by nurses and read by the attending physician. Some pediatricians became real experts in the field (see below) and usually were superior to the professional adult radiologists sent in later for help from the university centers. Initial interest was centered around the skeleton (rickets, scurvy, syphilis, osteomyelitis, trauma, etc.) and the chest (pneumonia, tuberculosis, etc.). Numerous papers from these institutions and from that time were illustrated with X-rays and concerned radiological subjects: The local history of pediatric radiology and a complete bibliography for Basel and Zurich is found in the two centenary books of these institutions (100 Jahre Kinderspital Basel 1962/Zürich 1974).

The History of Pediatric Radiology in Switzerland

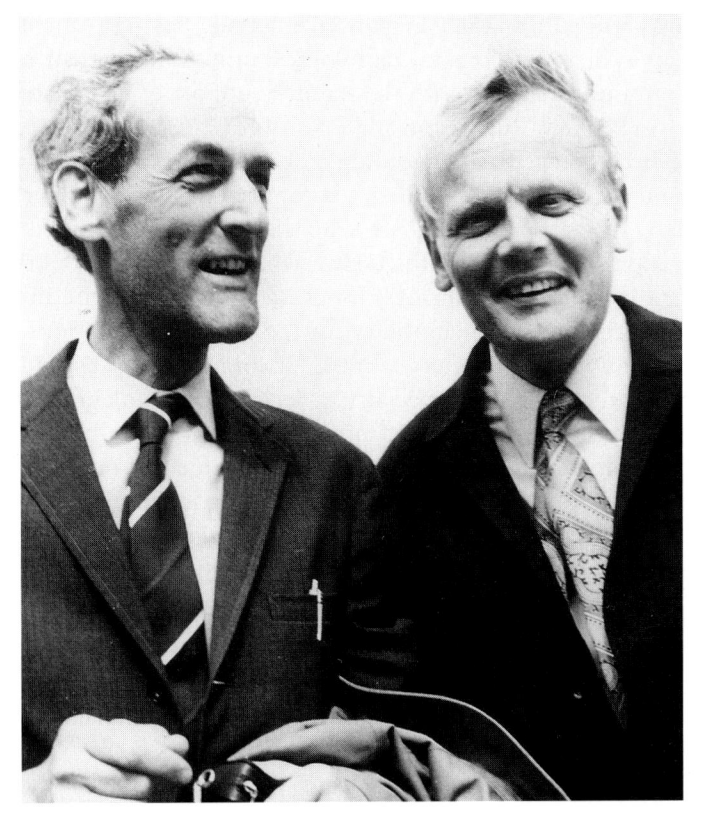

Figure 2
A. Giedion and K. D. Ebel during a moment of relaxation in 1970

Pediatric Radiology, the Illegitimate Child

During an after-dinner speech addressed to the ESPR members in Basel in 1967, Prof. F. Bamatter, head of the department of pediatrics at the University of Geneva and an ardent supporter of pediatric radiology, asked: "Why does the sullen father, radiology, not finally recognize his gorgeous and thriving child, issued from his union with the beautiful mother, pediatrics?" At that time, the Swiss Pediatric Society had already fully understood the importance of our field and considered its incorporation as a pediatric subspecialty. As indicated by Bamatter, the Swiss Radiological

Society was less enthusiastic, in particular about having "uncontrolled" activities away from the central radiological unit. With patient insistence, however, and in particular with the staunch support of far-sighted radiologists such as Prof. A. Rüttimann and Prof. W. Fuchs, we gradually reached our goal: In 1980, pediatric radiology became part of the Swiss board examination for diagnostic radiology, compulsory since 1988. The cases are provided by pediatric radiologists who also are the examiners of their specialty, and then selected by the board, which includes a pediatric radiologist. Since 1988, a minimum of 3 months' full-time practice in pediatric radiology is prerequisite to eligibility for the board examinations. In 1990, the Swiss Radiological Society almost unanimously accepted pediatric radiology as a recognized subspecialty, a decision that took effect in the fall of 1992. Finally, in recognition of our group's efforts on behalf of Swiss pediatric radiology, the writer of these lines became an honorary member of the Swiss Radiological Society in 1990. Pediatric radiology was chosen as the main topic at six annual meetings of the Swiss Radiological Society (Wieser), and twice by the Swiss Pediatric Society, including a joint meeting in 1946.

Societies of Pediatric Radiology in Switzerland, Europe and Worldwide

In 1978 the Swiss Society for Pediatric Radiology was founded by seven full-time pediatric radiologists. Heinz Tschäppeler was elected as our permanent secretary, Ulrich Willi, in 1992, as our first president. The European Society of Pediatric Radiology (ESPR) played a decisive role for Swiss pediatric radiology: Herbert Kaufmann, Daniel Nusslé, and I participated in the unforgettable *Réunion internationale de radiologie pédiatrique* in 1963 and the "first" ESPR meeting in 1964, where we became founding members, at the château de Longchamps near Paris. This society was, over the years, the "gold standard" for our own work, and a source of new information as well as of strength and confidence for our local efforts. Even more important, the ESPR created for all of us a worldwide, life-long net of personal friendships. On three occasions the ESPR met in Switzerland: In 1967 in Basel, Herbert Kaufmann's first 2-day post-congress tour turned out to be a particularly great success. He reminded us of the value of exchanging ideas outside the lecture hall. I regret that more recently, post-congress tours have tended to degenerate into simple travel-agency-organized multiple-choice items. In Lucerne in 1977 a first postgraduate course with original-scale X-ray copies for each participant was introduced by myself and a "philosophical" main topic, "problem-oriented pediatric radiology", was offered. In Montreux in 1988, Daniel Nusslé organized, for the first time in this society, a variety of excellent workshops and used an interdisciplinary approach to our problems. These meetings, to which the local authorities in radiology and pediatrics were always invited, greatly boosted the prestige of our specialty in Switzerland. It was considered a particular distinction for Swiss pediatric radiology that all three of us became honorary members of the ESPR and that one of us was chosen to deliver the Neuhauser lecture at the first joint meeting together with the SPR in Toronto 1987. The *"Gesellschaft für pädiatrische Radiologie (GPR)"* is discussed in another chapter. Herbert Kaufmann and I were among the founders. We received the society three times in Switzerland: myself, 1970 in Zurich; Chris Fliegel, 1982 in Basel; and Heinz Tschäppeler (HT), 1990 in Bern. HT and I were both members of the board. The positive effects of the GPR meetings on Swiss pediatric radiology were similar to those of the ESPR, though more intimate and on a smaller scale. One of our personal goals was to keep this society an international group of German-*speaking* pediatric radiologists from Austria, Holland, France (where German is also a native language!), at that time Western Germany and the German Democratic Republic, as well as from Switzerland, and to prevent it from turning into a strictly West German organization. For about 20 years now, a small, loosely organized group of 20–30 pediatric radiologists working in southern Germany, nearby France, Austria, and Switzerland, called the *"4-Länder-Klub"* (four-Country Club), has met twice a year for "family-reunion-like" film-reading sessions.

A Short History of the Eight Swiss Pediatric Radiology Units

There are four separate divisions or units of pediatric radiology in conjunction with the medical faculty of the respective universities of Switzerland. In Lausanne, as an exception, pediatric radiology is completely integrated in the university's adult radiology department, but two examination rooms are still reserved for pediatric patients. Otherwise, the head of pediatric radiology is appointed by the hospital and confirmed by the health department. One of his or her duties is to teach medical students weekly in small groups and to give a few formal lectures during the academic year. An academic degree may be obtained but is not a prerequisite for the position. So far, and to our regret, there is no formal academic chair for pediatric radiology in Switzerland. Depending on the geographical and historical circumstances, the connection between pediatric radiology and the university department of radiology varies from complete independence (Basel, Zurich) to partial integration (Geneva, Bern) and complete integration (Lausanne). There are three additional nonuniversity units of pediatric radiology in children's hospitals in the states (cantons) of Aargau (Aarau), Lucerne, and St. Gallen.

The following notes were compiled from data contributed by the present and/or former chief of each center and are acknowledged at the end of each section. Some information on workload and staff, as well as a list of the more sophisticated technical equipment *within* the division or unit is found in Tables 1 and 2. Examinations exceeding the possibilities of the individual center are carried out in the university department of radiology or state adult hospital.

Basel

In 1901, the first X-ray equipment was installed in the *Basler Kinderspital* (founded 1862). The choice of Prof. A. Hottinger 1954 as director of the department of pediatrics was favorable for the development of pediatric radiology, as he had shown an early and keen interest in this field. He was co-author of one of the first textbooks on pediatric radiology (Engel and Schall 1933). He encouraged and supported the emerging career of Herbert Kaufmann (HK), who in 1959, as a pediatric chief resident, was put in charge of the division of radiology. Already in 1958, when I was a fellow in E. B. D. Neuhauser's (EBDN) department of radiology in Boston, HK visited me and was impressed by this institution and its impact on pediatrics. During 1960 he also worked for 10 months as a fellow with EBDN. On returning to Basel in 1961, he continued his work in radiology, crowned in 1965 by his formal nomination as staff member and head (leitender Arzt) of the division of radiology, as well as (in 1963) by his academic promotion to assistent professor (*Privatdozent*) and (in 1970) associate professor at the university. HK was one of the founding members of the ESPR and president in 1967. In 1973, after HK had left for Philadelphia, Christian Fliegel (CHF), a former pediatrician, took over his position, after 2 years' training (1969–1971) with HK and 2 years (1972–1973) with EBDN in Boston. He is also a member of the ESPR. *Special fields of interest*: Orthopedic radiology, uroradiology of the newborn. *Data* from HK and CHF.

The History of Pediatric Radiology in Switzerland

Table 1
Medical and medical technical personnel in eight Swiss pediatric radiology units as of Dec. 31, 1991

	Pos. of Chief[a] Hosp./Acad.	Staff radiologist	Chief resident fellow	Regular resident	Rotating resident	Technicians
Aarau	2	1	–	–	1	1
Basel	2/ASSO	1	1	1	1	6
Bern	2/INST	1	–	–	1	5
Geneve	2/ASSI	1.2	1	–	1	7.5
Lausanne	2/INST	0.9	–	–	1	6
Lucerne	2	1	–	–	1	2
St. Gallen	2	1	–	–	1	4
Zurich	1/ASSI	2.6	1	1	1	8

[a] The position of the head of the unit may be equal to the other chiefs of a unit in the same hospital (1), like chief of anesthesia, etc. (*Chefarzt*), or one rank lower (2), usually under the medical director. The academic position may be that of an associate professor (ASSO), assistant professor (ASSI), or instructor (INST) at the medical school.

Table 2
Workload and special equipment in eight Swiss pediatric radiology units as of Dec. 31, 1991

	No. examinations (US) year	2 Plane angio.	Color doppler	Digit. fluor.	CT	MRI	Scintigraphy
Aarau	? (2 500)	–	–	–	–	–	–
Basel	12 500 (4 000)	+	+	–	–	–	–
Bern	16 000 (5 000)	–	+	–	–	–	–
Geneve	20 000 (3 000)	–	+	–	–	–	–
Lausanne[a]	14 000 (1 800)	+[a]	+[a]	+[a]	+[a]	+[a]	+[a]
Lucerne	8 470 (1 736)	–	–	–	–	–	–
St. Gallen	10 000 (4 500)	–	–	–	–	–	–
Zurich	23 000 (5 000)	+	–	+	+	+[b]	–

[a] Integrated into adult radiology department.
[b] Unit usable only for neonates and infants.

Bern

The *Jenner-Kinderspital* (founded in 1862) had no room for X-ray examinations when Prof. E. Rossi was elected in 1957 as new chief of pediatrics. Coming from the "Fanconi school" in Zurich, and an excellent radiologist himself, he was dismayed by the "level of this poor children's home equipped as for the year 1900." In the same year, Daniel Nusslé (DN), after 1 year of training at the university department for radiology in Lausanne, started as a *pediatric* resident under Rossi. In 1959, when two examination rooms were installed – one with amplified fluoroscopy, DN was put in charge of the GI and GU examinations, besides his other duties as a pediatrician on the ward. In 1961 DN left for Paris (see "Lausanne"), and in 1962 the Jenner Foundation was taken over by the University medical center, the *Inselspital Bern*. Thus, and in particular with the opening of a new children's hospital in 1978, also called the "Rossi Palace", with four X-ray examination rooms, pediatric radiology was increasingly taken over by the Central Department of Radiology, only 200 m distant. One of the radiological chief residents, Heinz Tschäppeler (HT), after an additional year each with Olle Eklöf (1974) at the Karolinska in Stockholm and with Fred Silverman (1975) in Cincinnati, became the first well-trained pediatric radiologist in Bern in 1976 and helped to plan the new department. This position was given a permanent staff status (leitender Arzt) in 1980, and in the same year HT became a full member of the ESPR. *Special fields of interest*: Pediatric uroradiology. *Data* from AG, DN, HT.

Geneva

The Geneva children's hospital (*clinique infantile*, founded in 1910) had its first conventional fluoroscopy unit installed only a few years before Prof. F. Bamatter 1957 became chairman of the department of pediatrics. In spite of strong opposition from the department of radiology, which objected to this "decentralization", and with only private funds, Bamatter opened a new examination room with a small image amplifier in 1958. The darkroom equipment had to be placed in the same room! He was assisted by Jean-Paul Rast, a trained radiologist, who at the time worked as pediatric resident in the department and thus became the first (part-time) pediatric radiologist. Later on, having left the hospital in 1959, Rast trained for 1 year with Jacques Lefèbvre in Paris, Ulf Rudhe in Stockholm, and Arnold Lassrich in Hamburg and became a member of the ESPR. Already in private practice, he supervised pediatric radiology as a consultant at the *clinique infantile* and participated in the design of the division of radiology, opened in 1961 in the new *clinique de pédiatrie*. But it was not until 1971, at the insistence of the new chairman of pediatrics, Prof. P. Ferrier, that a full-time position for a pediatric radiologist was created, occupied from the beginning by Daniel Nusslé. He also was given the academic title of "*chargé de cours en pédiatrie et radiologie pédiatrique*", in connection with his teaching of students and residents. The unit is integrated into the departments of radiology and pediatrics. The sabbaticals of G. Currarino, of H. Taybi, and (twice) of F. Silverman spent in DN's department were particular highlights of pediatric radiology in Geneva. *Special fields of interest*: GI and uroradiology. *Data* from DN.

Lausanne

When Daniel Nusslé (DN) arrived in Lausanne in 1963, the second station of his crusade for pediatric radiology, the *Clinique infantile*, founded in 1916, was in a condition similar to the one he had encountered first in Bern, with no room for X-ray examinations. In the meantime, DN had worked 1 year in the service of J. Lefèbvre in Paris and 4 months with U. Rudhe at the Karolinska in Stockholm. Still finishing his training in general radiology in the department of Prof. G. Candardjis, DN became "special full-time assistant in pediatric radiology," and was promoted in 1965 to staff member (*médecin adjoint*) for pediatric radiology. Typical for DNs "integrated" approach to medicine was his continued work as consultant in clinical pediatrics, in particular in pediatric gastroenterology. With great energy, finally under threat of resigning, and well supported by Prof. Jaccottet, chairman of pediatrics, DN installed a pediatric radiology unit *within* the *clinique infantile*, similar to the "new" one of Bern, which was opened in 1965. Michel Bugnion, at that time chief resident in radiology, with his great interest in GI studies in infants, and in particular with his excellent cine-radiographic studies on deglutition and gastroesophageal reflux, had already broken the ground for this development. The new service worked very well, but eventually the central department felt uneasy about the (too) strong integration of "its" branch into pediatrics, leading in 1971 to the departure of DN for Geneva. In 1980, the building of the *Centre Hospitalier Universitaire Vaudois* (CHUV) was completed. This big complex contains the pediatric and pediatric-surgical departments as well as the university department of radiology, where two examination rooms are reserved exclusively for pediatric patients. Uniquely for a modern Swiss university center, pediatric radiology was now done on a part-time basis by two radiologists trained in pediatric radiology, J. Queloz (member of the ESPR) and M. Landry. In 1988, Dr. F. Gudinchet (FG) became head (*médecin associé*) of the "integrated" unit of pediatric radiology. After his training as a radiologist he had worked for 1 year with Denis Lallemand at the *Hôpital des Enfants Malades* in Paris, and he became a member of the ESPR 1989. *Special field of interest*: MRI. *Data* from FG and DN.

Zurich

The first room for X-ray examinations at the *Kinderspital* (founded in 1874) was installed in 1904. Under Guido Fanconi, head of the department of pediatrics from 1929 to 1962 and one of the towering universal pediatricians of this century, the hospital became an internationally known center of pediatric care and research. Fanconi was also a brilliant interpreter of X-ray images. He considered the contribution of radiology to the development of pediatrics to be as important as that of biochemistry (Giedion 1974). During my 3 years of *pediatric* training at the Children's Hospital Medical Center in Boston (1951–1954) I observed daily the most substantial, for me sometimes miraculous, contributions of Dr. E. B. D. Neuhauser (EBDN) and his crew to the solution of our diagnostic problems. Back in Zurich, as a resident in Fanconi's department, our radiology seemed to be medieval. Fanconi understood me at once, and allowed me to work for a year in the adult radiology department of H. R. Schinz, while still covering the radiology unit at the children's hospital. After I had severed an additional fellowship of 14 months with EBDN in 1958/1959, he called me back urgently to start as a full-time pediatric radiologist on June 1st, 1959. Slowly climbing the hierarchic ladder, I finally received the position of *Chefarzt*, head of the division of radiology in 1978. The importance of this hospital status, unique in Swiss pediatric radiology, but standard in adult radiology, cannot be overestimated, in particular when one is bargaining directly with the health department. It carries more practical weight than an academic position (I became assistant professor in 1976) and marks the end of pediatric radiology being an "illegitimate child". Initially, things moved slowly, however: After my return Prof. Max Grob, the pioneer of Swiss pediatric surgery and an expert interpreter of radiographs, bluntly told me: "I do my radiology and you do yours," which restricted me to nonsurgical cases. Yet a few days later, I was called to advise in a case of H-type fistula which had escaped diagnostic demonstration by Grob himself, the adult radiology department, and the adult ENT service. In a few minutes, with my "Boston technique", the high fistula at C-5 was demonstrated. Grob was thrilled when I proposed an approach from the neck, thus avoiding thoracotomy, and said: "Now you may also do *my* radiology," and also suggested a publication of the case (Giedion 1960). We became good friends. In 1969 a new wing of our hospital was built including a modern radiology division with five examination rooms according to my design. My fight for a CT unit beginning in 1982 became successful only at the end of my carrier, through a spectacular deal with the department of health, worthy of being copied: As we are a tertiary care center for trauma cases, including those of the head, a CT within the hospital was an absolute necessity. However, we were not able to produce the yearly number of 2400 CT examinations required by the government. Finally, an ingenious solution was found: The adult central radiology department would send us the missing 1200 cases, thus diminishing their own waiting list. Such a deal of course requires an understanding, broad-minded "adult" counterpart; in our case this was Prof. W. Fuchs, at the university radiology department. Happily, 1 ½ years after my retirement in 1990, my successor Ulrich Willi (UW) was able to inaugurate "our" CT. UW, pediatrician and radiologist alike, trained in pediatric radiology first with me and then 3 years with John Kirkpatrick, thus representing the second Bostonian generation in our division. He also is a member of the ESPR. Finally, the MRI unit as a part of imaging in our hospital, yet not belonging to "our" radiology, should be mentioned: Originally planned by the group of Dr. E. Martin and colleagues as a tool for MR spectroscopy, their 2.35-Tesla magnet with a boreheole of only 40 cm and with their ingenious devices for the examination of artificially ventilated babies turned out to be an excellent instrument for the imaging of the brain of small infants (Boesch and Martin 1988, Martin et al. 1990). *Special fields of interest*: Pediatric urology, genetic bone disease. *Data* from AG.

The *three nonuniversity units of pediatric radiology* were opened simultaneously with the newly established children's hospitals in Aarau (1955), St. Gallen (1966), and Lucerne (1972). Each has two examination rooms, one equipped with fluoroscopy, and they are run by a full-time pediatric radiologist: The late Marco Brandner was the first head (1970–1972) in Aarau, followed by Marcus Wita (1977–1991). The present head, since 1992, is Elke Schaefer (ES), a former staff member from the radiological division of the children's hospital of Altona and member of the ESPR. Roger Kwasny (RK) has been the head in Lucerne since 1977, Dr. Peter Waibel (PW) the head in St. Gallen since 1985. The latter two have trained with Heinz Tschäppeler in Bern, and all three have the status of a staff member (*leitender Arzt*). *Data* from RK, ES and PW.

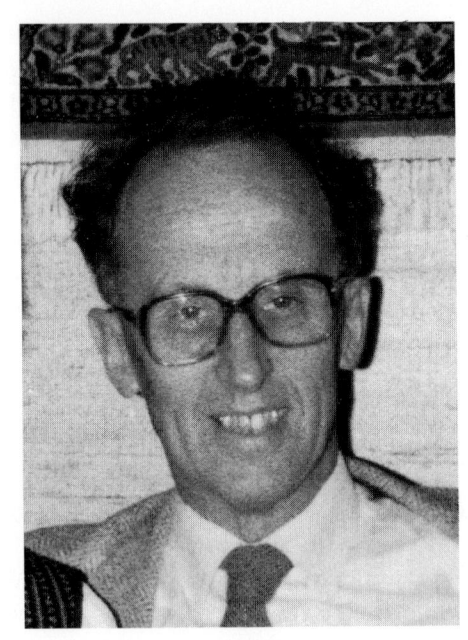

Figure 3
Dr. Daniel Nusslé, Geneva (1987)

References

Boesch C, Martin E (1988) Combined application of MR imaging and spectroscopy in neonates and children: installation and operation of a 2.35-T system in a clinical setting. Radiology 168:481–488
Engel S, Schall L (1933) Handbuch der Röntgendiagnostik und -Therapie im Kindesalter. Thieme, Leipzig
Giedion A (1960) Angeborene hohe Oesophagotrachealfistel vom H-Typus. Helv Paed Acta 15:155–162
Giedion A (1974) Radiologie. In: 100 Jahre Kinderspital Zürich, p 95
100 Jahre Kinderspital in Basel 1862–1962. 1962 Kinderspital Basel
100 Jahre Kinderspital Zürich 1874–1974. 1974 Kinderspital Zürich
Kaufmann HJ (1962) Historisches über die Anfänge der Röntgendiagnostik am Basler Kinderspital. Annales Paediatrici 199:175–186
Wieser C (1989) Von den Anfängen der Radiologie in der Schweiz. In: Wieser C, Etter H, Wellauer J (eds) Radiologie in der Schweiz. Huber, Bern, p 19

Springer-Verlag and the Environment

We at Springer-Verlag firmly believe that an international science publisher has a special obligation to the environment, and our corporate policies consistently reflect this conviction.

We also expect our business partners – paper mills, printers, packaging manufacturers, etc. – to commit themselves to using environmentally friendly materials and production processes.

The paper in this book is made from low- or no-chlorine pulp and is acid free, in conformance with international standards for paper permanency.